The Lupus Cookbook

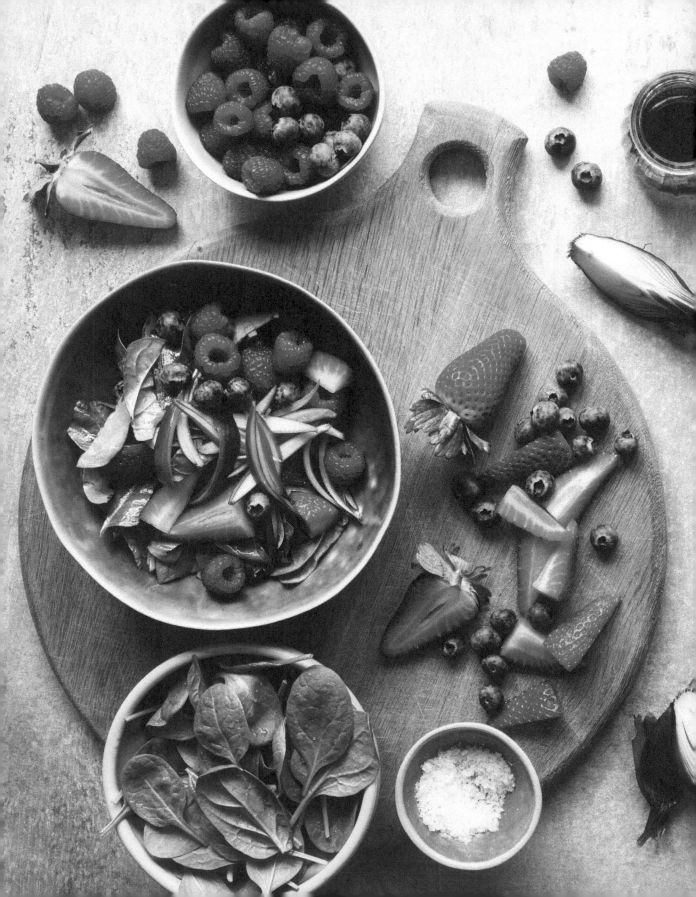

The
LUPUS
COOKBOOK

125+ Anti-Inflammatory Recipes to Live Well with Lupus

Ana Reisdorf, MS, RD

Foreword by Jeanette Alston-Watkins
of Lupus Foundation of America

Photography by Nadine Greeff

ROCKRIDGE
PRESS

For general information on our other products and services or to obtain technical support, please contact our Customer Care Department within the United States at (866) 744-2665, or outside the United States at (510) 253-0500.

Rockridge Press publishes its books in a variety of electronic and print formats. Some content that appears in print may not be available in electronic books, and vice versa.

Cover Designer: Amy King
Photo Art Director: Amy Hartmann
Editor: Salwa Jabado
Production Editor: Andrew Yackira
Photography © Nadine Greeff, 2018.
Author photo © Kaysha Weiner
www.kayshaweiner.com, 2018.

ISBN: Print 978-1-64152-243-4 | eBook 978-1-64152-244-1
R1

This book is for the lupus sufferer who is without hope, who is looking for a solution, who wants to achieve true health and well-being.

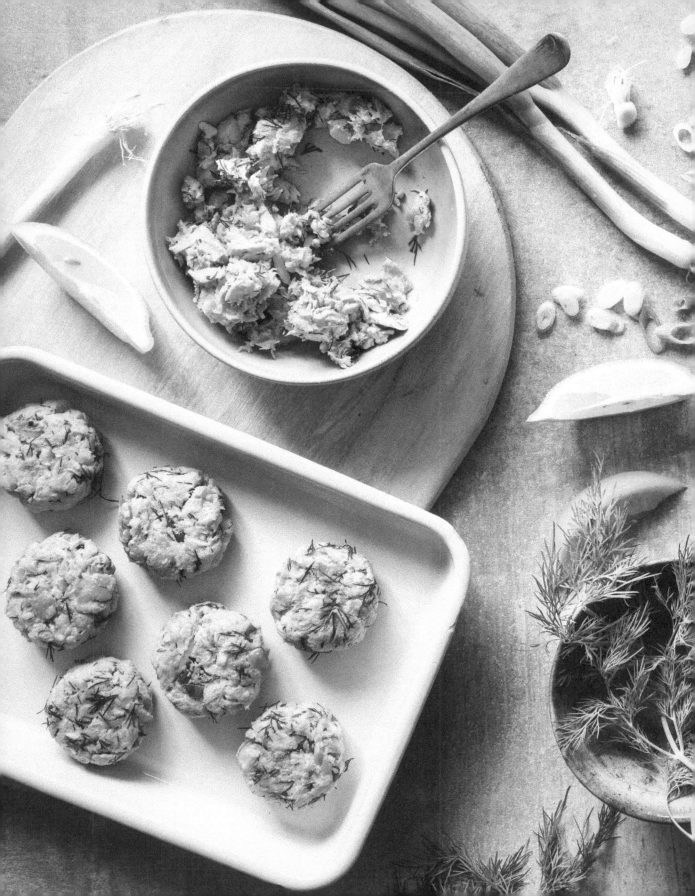

Contents

Foreword

The Lupus Cookbook is an investment in your future health. If you've been diagnosed with lupus or any autoimmune disease, you realize your life needs to change. Like most people, you may be wondering where to start—but you're already in the right place. Being diagnosed with a disease that has no cure is a shock to the system. Even though it can't be cured, you have the power to put it into remission. Yes, you read that correctly—*you have the power*. *The Lupus Cookbook* makes it easy for anyone to follow the recipes and make an amazing meal even on days when you don't feel like you're capable of doing anything. I wish these recipes were around over ten years ago when I first found out I had lupus. I might have cooked more.

I've lived with lupus, fibromyalgia, Raynaud's, Sjögren syndrome, and a few other autoimmune issues for over ten years while juggling a full-time job and a family. I was taking thirty-six pills a day and a Benlysta infusion once a month, and still had some aches and pains and felt totally fatigued. I was never hospitalized due to lupus, but I had my share of horrible days that included debilitating pain, paralysis, inflammation, infections, and Plaquenil toxicity. I needed to do something before I ended up having organ issues due to all the medication I was on.

I would ask doctors and others, "Can a change in diet help patients with lupus?" I was told, "No, there's really nothing out there," or "Try to eat a healthier diet." What exactly did that mean? That's when I started paying close attention to what my body was telling me, and took my diet into my own hands. I started logging my food intake. I started to notice how some of my favorite foods were causing me some issues ranging from stomach pains to full inflammation. I noticed that, once I eliminated sugar, my brain fog, fatigue, and pain were reduced and eventually subsided entirely. Then I began eliminating other foods like eggplant, bean sprouts, and alfalfa, which had been causing me stomachaches, joint pain, and inflammation. Finally,

I realized that most of these are nightshades and known foods that lupus patients shouldn't eat. I knew I had to make a huge change to my diet if I wanted a better quality of life. *The Lupus Cookbook* takes all that work out of meal planning for you.

The Lupus Cookbook is exactly what I was looking for so many years ago. Ana Reisdorf carefully explains why certain foods worsen inflammation for us and gives us the information we need in order to understand why we shouldn't eat something and may want to substitute it for something else. My favorite part is the Lupus-Friendly Kitchen Staples. Don't you hate it when you're about to start cooking an amazing meal and realize that you forgot something? This section helps us novices in the kitchen become experts. Another great tool is the recipe labels listing what you might need that day, or what you might need due to other diseases—Flare Soother, Fatigue-Friendly, Kidney Support, Cardio Care, and Bone Booster. You will know exactly where to go for recipes to support your lupus journey.

With *The Lupus Cookbook*, I now have an arsenal of good, solid meals that I can fall back on so that I'll never get bored. It's never too late to start something new that can help you or a loved one live a very long, pain-free life.

If diet can bring back my eyesight and my health without medication, don't you think you should consider what you eat? Diet and nutrition are so important in managing lupus and autoimmune diseases. If it can help keep me off medication, it might be able to help you reduce your medication or prevent some of the damage that some of the medication may cause.

ABOUT THE FOREWORD WRITER

Jeanette Alston-Watkins is the Lupus Ambassador, Facilitator, and Advocate for the Lupus Foundation of America, Florida Chapter. She was the 2018 Team Advisor for PatientsLikeMe.com. She has been a Lupus Warrior for over 10 years, is an upcoming author, and a Lupus Life Coach. She dedicates her time to helping newly diagnosed patients understand that they are not alone, and guides lupus and other autoimmune patients in the right direction. She feels blessed in knowing that God had a plan for her in helping others through this disease.

Introduction

As a registered dietitian (RD), I have been trained to first look at diet as a way to manage symptoms of any illnesses and to help people feel better. Even if a diet change doesn't cure a disease, choosing healthy food will always improve your health.

About 10 years ago, I had some weird unexplained symptoms—joint pain, fatigue. After many doctor appointments and medical tests, my rheumatologist told me I had an autoimmune disease, but he just couldn't pinpoint which one, maybe lupus, maybe something else.

Being an RD, I immediately went online to research how I could change my diet to improve my symptoms. Sadly, I found nothing. All the websites for autoimmune diseases said to "eat a healthy diet." There were no specifics available. But I kept digging. Eventually, I came across a doctor who recommended I eliminate grains and sugar from my diet. Within three days my joint pain was gone. I followed an anti-inflammatory diet, as outlined in this book, for a long time, and my symptoms never returned.

During this same time, in my practice I kept seeing patients who were looking for answers for their own autoimmune conditions. Their search had resulted in the same thing—little to no information on how to manage their illness with diet. Through my own personal and professional experience, I was able to guide them to follow a similar protocol to the one I had used, and their symptoms visibly improved. I was able to make them feel better through diet.

Sadly, rates of autoimmune diseases are skyrocketing. The answer in the medical community seems to be more and stronger medications to help control the immune system. Although these medications work relatively well, many have very serious side effects. Most doctors rarely mention diet and lifestyle changes as alternatives for addressing autoimmune conditions.

In these modern times, we are lucky that medical advances have dramatically improved the ability of people to live well with autoimmune diseases such as lupus. But medications should not be seen as the only option to help manage this condition. Other lifestyle interventions, including diet, can really make an impact.

Lupus can be debilitating; the fatigue can be completely draining, making even the simplest tasks almost impossible to complete. So why not give people more natural options to manage flares and inflammation?

Luckily, there is more and more research being done on diet changes to improve autoimmune disease symptoms. Lupus sufferers who want to change their diet to help manage their symptoms no longer lack resources. With the internet, there may now even be too much information, with an almost-overwhelming deluge of discussions about how to eat an anti-inflammatory diet. Some of the advice is credible, while some of it is not. Regardless, how could someone with lupus not be intrigued and want to know more?

You want a source you can trust. As an RD, I completely understand that research-based recommendations are very important. And you also need practical information about exactly what to eat This book was designed to provide tasty, easy to make, anti-inflammatory recipes using current evidence-based recommendations to help manage common symptoms of lupus.

There is no cure for lupus, but that doesn't mean there can't be any hope. While an anti-inflammatory diet won't take away every symptom, there is no denying the powerful effects of certain foods on your health. Food is energy, and eating the right high-quality food can mean the difference between sickness and wellness.

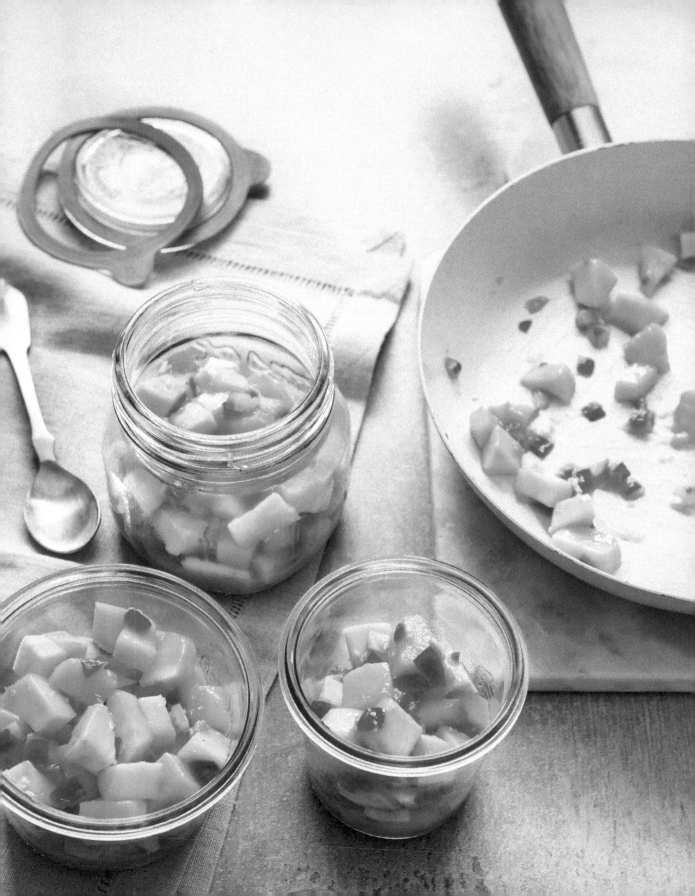

1

Lupus and Diet

Lupus is an autoimmune disease that can damage almost any part of the body. The word "lupus" usually refers to systemic lupus erythematosus (SLE), but there are several other kinds of lupus, differentiated by the area of the body affected by the disease. Regardless of the specific type, lupus is a chronic illness, meaning it can last for many years. It has no known cure.

Lupus symptoms are caused by the immune system attacking the body's healthy tissues and organs. Depending on where the attack happens, this can lead to significant inflammation, pain, and destruction of healthy organs. Lupus is usually diagnosed in people ages 15 to 44 and is more common in women. The severity of lupus can vary, ranging from mild to life-threatening.

Lupus can be a scary diagnosis to receive. But there is hope. Diet and lifestyle changes can help not only manage symptoms and flares but may also be able to send lupus into remission. Although you can never be cured of lupus, by taking care of yourself you can usually live a long, fulfilling, and healthy life.

Facing page: Mango Chutney, page 159

1

Eating for Health

Whether you were just diagnosed with lupus or you have had it for a while, it's never too late to start thinking about what you eat and how it affects your health. You probably already know that a good diet is fundamental to your overall well-being and one of the best ways to take care of yourself, whether you have lupus or not.

With any way of eating, there is no one size fits all. It's true that there is no conclusive evidence that points to one particular diet that will completely eradicate lupus for everyone. And such a diet may never exist, because humans are complex beings. How well a diet works for a person with a particular disease depends on genetics, the severity of the disease itself, stress, and myriad other lifestyle factors that are difficult to control. However, a healthy diet will always be one major factor in making you feel better.

This book and the recipes in it are based on the current research available about lupus, inflammation, and diet. Since lupus is an autoimmune disease, one of its major underlying triggers is inflammation. If you have lupus, you have likely felt the adverse effects of inflammation—joint pain, fatigue, or skin rashes. All of these are symptoms of the inflammation that occurs when the immune system goes rogue and starts attacking the body's own healthy tissues.

It is widely agreed that some foods trigger inflammation, while others are anti-inflammatory. But trying to figure out which foods are best to eat for lupus by researching online can be extremely confusing and overwhelming. The information can be totally contradictory.

This book was written to give you some specific ideas of what to eat to help manage this chronic illness. Lupus does not affect everyone in the same way, but the goal is to get you on the path to feeling better. The recipes are loaded with anti-inflammatory foods to reduce two of the most debilitating lupus symptoms, pain and fatigue.

The other goal of this book is to give you easy and delicious recipes, so you know exactly what to eat. When you are struggling with a lupus flare, the last thing you need is to spend hours in the kitchen. Keeping it simple and easy is vitally important when you are struggling with low energy. The autoimmune diet can be quite restrictive, so it is important for the recipes to be tasty, making it easier to stick with the protocol. This recipe book was written with you in mind, to help you take control of one of the most important factors in your health and well-being: your diet.

The Diet Connection

Diet is one of the main influencers of how you feel, particularly when you have been diagnosed with a chronic disease. But diet is only one part of what should be a multipronged approach to health and well-being. Other pieces of the puzzle to help you live better with lupus may include medication, exercise, stress management, quality sleep, and mental health.

This book focuses only on food, because changing your diet is a great first step toward feeling better—and also because you eat multiple times a day! But to truly send lupus into remission, you will likely have to address those other lifestyle aspects as well.

Since this is a cookbook, however, let's focus on diet. What are the guidelines for managing lupus symptoms? The diet outlined in this book is based on what is commonly referred to as the autoimmune protocol, or AIP. This is a modified version of the Paleo or caveman diet, which many people are familiar with. The AIP was designed to address four specific areas, helping manage triggers and symptoms of this illness.

GOAL: RESTORE GUT HEALTH

One trigger of autoimmune diseases is poor gut health. This can include an imbalance of healthy microbes in the digestive tract, leading to what is called dysbiosis or bacterial overgrowth. When there are too many of the bad bacteria in the gut, this triggers inflammation by signaling the immune system to react. One of the goals of the AIP diet is to help restore balance in the intestinal flora.

Many people with lupus also have a condition called leaky gut or increased intestinal permeability. This occurs when the spaces between intestinal cells get damaged, allowing food molecules, viruses, and bacteria to pass through unchecked. When this happens, the immune cells that sit outside the gut begin to attack those unexpected substances. The problem is that many of these substances look quite similar to the body's own cells and tissues. Unable to tell friend from foe, the immune system has mounted an attack against the body itself, leading to an autoimmune disease and chronic inflammation.

Balancing the gut microbes and repairing leaky gut are two of the primary goals of the AIP diet. Healing the digestive system is the first step toward lowering inflammation and improving symptoms.

GOAL: REDUCE INFLAMMATION

Inflammation is a natural process of the immune system that helps the body heal itself after an injury. Everyone has experienced inflammation at some point. For example, when you have a small cut, the body jumps into action right away to heal the injury. You may feel a bit of swelling, warmth, and redness in the area for a few days. That feeling is inflammation, the body working to repair itself. This is an incredible and helpful process, when it works well.

But in our current environment we are constantly exposed to many triggers causing inflammation: poor diet, toxins, smoking, stress, and pollution, among others. The body is always reacting to these triggers, leading to a constant, chronic state of inflammation. When the immune cells are always active, they start to attack the body's own tissues. This is when autoimmune diseases occur. The location of the attack usually determines the type of disease. So a diet to help control symptoms of lupus must also help reduce inflammation, one of the major underlying triggers of autoimmune diseases.

GOAL: INCREASE NUTRIENT DENSITY

Your body, which includes your immune system, requires vitamins, minerals, protein, healthy fats, and antioxidants to function correctly. Nutrient deficiencies can trigger inflammation and the development of autoimmune diseases such as lupus. A nutrient-dense diet can help correct these deficiencies, support a strong immune system, and help reduce inflammation. The AIP is a diet high in the nutrients required for optimal health, supporting the body in repairing damaged tissues.

GOAL: BALANCE HORMONES

Hormones are chemical signalers that control everything from how the immune system works to how we feel day to day. Hormones play a major role in the development of autoimmune diseases, although the relationship is complex and still not well understood.

Women in particular are at greater risk of developing autoimmune diseases, particularly during their reproductive years. An imbalance of the hormone estrogen may play a role, because levels are higher during that time in a woman's life. Estrogen is known to trigger inflammation.

Lupus in particular is very hormone-sensitive, which is why it is seen more often in women. Hormonal birth control pills and hormone replacement therapy have been shown to increase the likelihood of developing lupus, particularly for those who have a genetic predisposition.

The AIP diet is meant to help balance hormones, reduce inflammation and manage lupus symptoms.

Five Steps to Managing Symptoms with an Anti-Inflammatory Diet

To keep things simple so you can get started right away, here are some very basic guidelines to follow for an anti-inflammatory diet.

1. **Base all your meals and snacks on anti-inflammatory foods.** If the goal is to lower inflammation, your diet will have to be based mostly on anti-inflammatory foods. These will include a diet full of healthy fats, colorful vegetables, and protein.

2. **Eat whole foods. Avoid processed foods.** Processed foods tend to be full of chemicals and devoid of any real nutrition. They do not support the body's need for real, whole nutrients. The basis of the AIP is to provide the body with high-quality nutrition, which simply cannot be found in most processed foods.

3. **Avoid highly inflammatory foods such as grains, dairy, and sugar.** Grains should be completely avoided on the AIP diet, particularly those containing gluten, such as wheat, barley, and rye. Gluten is a trigger for leaky gut and inflammation. Dairy is inflammatory in two ways. First, a protein in dairy called casein is quite similar in structure to gluten, making it highly inflammatory. Additionally, many people are sensitive to the sugar in dairy, called lactose. Lactose intolerance can lead to gas, bloating, and diarrhea, all of which can make leaky gut worse. Sugar is very inflammatory and should be avoided completely.

THE MEDICINE-DIET RELATIONSHIP

Lupus is frequently managed either with medications that suppress the immune system—to prevent it overreacting and attacking the body—or with anti-inflammatory medications. Many of these medications work quite well to manage symptoms and can be part of a well-rounded treatment plan for lupus. But many of them can have very serious side effects—discuss details with a doctor before starting treatment.

Common medications used to treat lupus include the following:

- Steroids or glucocorticoids, such as prednisone
- Chemotherapy agents, such as methotrexate
- Cytokine blockers, such as Humira and Enbrel
- Nonsteroidal anti-inflammatory medications (NSAIDs), such as ibuprofen
- Pain medications

If you take any of these medications, here are some tips for making better food choices.

Steroids: These can increase your appetite significantly and lead to weight gain. Try to manage your weight by choosing healthy but filling low-calorie foods to snack on, such as fruits and vegetables. A higher protein diet is usually recommended to help counteract some of the side effects. Choose foods low in sodium but high in magnesium, potassium, and calcium, as steroids tend to deplete these minerals. Increase your exercise to try to counteract some of these effects.

Chemotherapy agents: Methotrexate in particular can deplete the body of folate, an important vitamin for DNA synthesis and cell replication. If you are taking this medication, it is important to supplement with folate and eat foods high in this B vitamin, such as green leafy vegetables.

NSAIDs: These medications can alter the natural gut flora and trigger leaky gut, making inflammation worse long-term. Regularly eating fermented foods or taking probiotics can help manage some of these side effects.

Pain medications: A common side effect of pain medications, particularly narcotics, is constipation. Increase your water and fiber intake to try to improve symptoms. You can also try an over-the-counter psyllium supplement.

4. **Avoid inflammatory fats, such as certain polyunsaturated fats and trans fats.** While some polyunsaturated fats, such as the omega-3s, are anti-inflammatory, others are highly inflammatory—specifically, certain omega-6 fats, such as vegetable oil. Omega-6 fats also interfere with the absorption of the anti-inflammatory omega-3s. Trans fats are industrially made fats that have been linked to inflammation and an increased risk for several diseases. The FDA banned them completely in June of 2018, but food manufacturers do not have to comply until 2020. These are mostly found in packaged foods because they increase shelf stability.

5. **Avoid alcohol.** The breakdown of alcohol releases a toxic compound called acetaldehyde, which is highly inflammatory. It is a known carcinogen, damaging cells and forming free radicals in the body. People with lupus should limit or avoid alcohol completely, as it can be a major trigger for flares and pain.

Foods that Fight Inflammation

What should you eat to fight inflammation? Many of the foods included in this list won't be a surprise to you. Fruits, vegetables, and healthy fats and proteins make up the bulk of what is included in the AIP diet. They are grouped below by food group, so you can quickly make choices from each category when planning meals. Basing your diet on these anti-inflammatory choices, while avoiding inflammatory foods, will help reduce pain and fatigue, improving your well-being.

MEAT AND PROTEINS

The AIP includes almost all fresh, unprocessed meat, fish, poultry, and organ meats. Always choose the highest quality possible. Ideally, all your meat should be antibiotic-free and hormone-free, organic, and grass-fed or pasture-raised.

For fish, choose those highest in omega-3s, the highly anti-inflammatory fats. These are usually fatty, wild-caught fish. Avoid farm-raised fish, which are low in omega-3s. The Environmental Working Group maintains a Seafood Guide on its website (ewg.org/research/ewgs-good-seafood-guide# .W14wG34nbm0) listing the fish highest in omega-3s and lowest in mercury, a brain toxin.

A PLANT-BASED DIET

You may notice that the anti-inflammatory diet is heavily plant-based. Although it does include animal protein as the primary protein source, the majority of the foods allowed on the diet are plants. Plants are bursting with antioxidants, making them incredibly beneficial and anti-inflammatory, which is why there's a whole chapter of plant-based recipes in this book. There is some major power in plants!

Plant proteins, such as beans and tofu, are not allowed in the AIP due to their antinutrient and lectin content. Antinutrients are plant compounds that interfere with the body's ability to absorb many vitamins and minerals. Lectins are one of these antinutrients that have been shown to be particularly problematic for people struggling with inflammation. These plant compounds are hard to digest and can worsen leaky gut syndrome and trigger inflammation.

You may wonder why animal protein is included, since it has long been vilified in the nutrition community. With a few exceptions, animal protein is not inflammatory and actually provides several important nutrients difficult to find elsewhere. When lean meat replaces refined carbohydrates in the diet, inflammation decreases. Additionally, fish is high in omega-3 fats, which are highly anti-inflammatory. So although the diet for managing lupus should be mostly plant-based to help manage symptoms, there is no need to exclude animal protein.

FRUITS AND VEGETABLES

All vegetables are included, with the exception of those in the nightshade category, which will be discussed in the next section. Choose a variety of vegetables daily. You may have heard you should "eat the rainbow": red, white, orange/yellow, green, and purple. This is because each of these colors means the food contains a different nutrient and antioxidant. Eating a variety of vegetables is the best way to ensure you are getting all the nutrition you need. Aim for at least five servings of vegetables daily.

Fruit is incredibly healthy and full of vitamins and minerals, but it is high in sugar. Although the sugar in fruit is naturally occurring, too much can trigger inflammation in some people. Limit your servings of fruit to no more than two a day. Choose fruits that are low on the glycemic index. The glycemic index is a scale that measures how much a food affects your blood sugar level. In general, fruits low on the glycemic index include berries, cherries, apples, pears, citrus fruits, and stone fruits such as peaches and plums.

White potatoes are not allowed on the AIP, since they are part of the nightshade family, but sweet potatoes and other tubers are. Feel free to include these in your diet as a healthy source of complex carbohydrates.

HEALTHY FATS

Many of the common cooking fats we use are highly inflammatory. Fats to choose for cooking include coconut oil, avocado oil, and olive oil. Consuming avocados is also encouraged.

SPICES AND CONDIMENTS

We all want our food to taste good! Spices and condiments that are allowed on the diet include fresh or dried herbs and vinegar. Salt and black pepper are allowed for flavor. For adding sweetness, you can use small amounts of honey, real maple syrup, or coconut sugar.

You'll notice that the recipes in this book call for sea salt. Sea salt is a minimally processed salt made from evaporated salt water. It is rich in minerals and typically does not contain additives to prevent clumping, as table salt does. It is also slightly higher in some minerals than regular salt, but has no added iodine and therefore won't affect the thyroid. Because many autoimmune diseases show up together, it's not uncommon for someone with

FERMENTED FOODS AND INFLAMMATION

Fermented foods are foods that contain healthy bacteria and help create and maintain a healthy digestive tract. As we have discussed, bacterial imbalance in the gut can trigger inflammation. The bad bacteria send signals to the immune system, causing it to attack. Therefore, it is critical to keep these bad microbes in check by having plenty of good ones in the gut.

The recipes in this book include many fermented foods that you can make at home, if you are feeling motivated to do so. If not, it's perfectly okay to buy them at the store. Here is a short list of the most beneficial fermented foods for lupus that you can incorporate into your diet.

- Sauerkraut

- Water kefir

- Coconut kefir

- Kombucha

- Coconut milk yogurt

- White kimchi (does not contain nightshades)

- Fermented vegetables: beets, carrots, cauliflower, okra, etc.

- Pickles or fermented cucumbers

Select a few of your favorites and try to eat one or more daily. Eating fermented foods is recommended over taking a probiotic, because ferments contain a greater variety of bacterial strands than can be found in a pill, leading to an even healthier gut.

lupus to also have thyroid issues. Look for unrefined sea salt that does not contain any additives (read the labels!) at your local grocery store or health food store.

BEVERAGES

Water is always the best beverage. Herbal, green, and black teas are also allowed.

Foods that Worsen Inflammation

To lower inflammation, you must not only eat anti-inflammatory foods but also avoid inflammatory foods. There may be a few that surprise you on this "do not eat" list, but they are there because they are known gut irritants that trigger inflammation in people with autoimmune diseases, even if they are considered healthy foods for other people.

To see major changes in your symptoms, you must completely eliminate these foods from your diet for at least six weeks. You may be able to reintroduce some of them into your diet later, but some you may never be able to eat again without triggering a flare.

EGGS AND PLANT PROTEINS

The main source of protein on the AIP is animal protein, with one exception—eggs. It is important to avoid eggs, particularly egg whites. The protein in eggs is highly allergenic and is known to pass through the gut wall undigested, leading to an immune response. For people who do not have an autoimmune disease, this is not a problem, but people with lupus are much more sensitive to these proteins and the inflammation triggered by their presence.

You should also avoid plant proteins, such as beans and tofu, due to their saponin content. Saponins can enter the blood stream, triggering immune cells to initiate an inflammatory response. This is usually not a problem for most people, but those with autoimmune diseases can be sensitive to the action of these plant compounds.

GRAINS AND STARCHES

Avoid all grains and starches on the AIP. Those that are particularly problematic for the digestive tract and cause inflammation are foods made with wheat. Anything made with wheat (including wheat varieties such as spelt, kamut, faro, and durum, plus products such as bulgur and semolina), barley, rye, and triticale contains the protein gluten. Oats can be contaminated with gluten, and some people react to oats in a similar way as they do to wheat, so it is best to avoid them. Gluten has been found to be a trigger for leaky gut and other types of inflammation. Other grains, such as rice and quinoa, also have inflammatory properties and should be avoided.

NIGHTSHADE FRUIT AND VEGETABLES

There is a particular class of fruits and vegetables called the nightshades, and they are considered by many to be triggers for autoimmune diseases. Nightshades include white potatoes, tomatoes, eggplant, okra, hot peppers, sweet (bell) peppers, tomatillos, sorrel, cape gooseberries, ground cherries, pepino melons, paprika, cayenne pepper, capsicum, and goji berries.

DAIRY

People with autoimmune diseases are particularly sensitive to dairy products. Not only does cow's milk contain many allergens, but the protein in dairy, called casein, is similar in structure to gluten. Casein can have the same inflammatory effects as gluten. In addition, lactose, the sugar found in dairy, can cause digestive problems for those who are lactose intolerant. This can irritate a sensitive gut even further and lead to a variety of symptoms such as bloating, diarrhea, and gas.

SUGAR AND NON-NUTRITIVE SWEETENERS

The only sweeteners allowed on the AIP are honey, coconut sugar, and real maple syrup, in very small quantities. You must avoid sugar, agave syrup, and sugar substitutes. Sugar is in almost every packaged food as an additive. Sugar promotes inflammation, and you may find that when you overdo it with sugar, it leads to a flare-up. Artificial sweeteners can lead to elevated insulin levels, and many people with autoimmune diseases are sensitive to this.

FOOD ADDITIVES

Food additives are found in processed foods under many different names. There are more than 3,000 food additives that the FDA allows in our food. Many of these are common substances, such as salt, but many are more complex chemicals and artificial flavors. These additives are allowed in our food because they are considered by the FDA to be "generally recognized as safe" or GRAS. The words "generally recognized" don't give me much faith in the safety of these additives.

The problem is not so much each additive individually, but how they might interact with one another. These interactions are something we know very little about, so for people with autoimmune diseases, it is best to avoid processed foods entirely.

NUTS AND SEEDS

Nuts and seeds are common allergens and can trigger the immune system to respond in people who are particularly sensitive, such as those with lupus. Therefore, it is best to avoid nuts and seeds when you are trying to send lupus into remission.

ALCOHOL AND COFFEE

As we have discussed, the breakdown of alcohol releases a toxic chemical that promotes inflammation and the formation of free radicals. It should be significantly limited or avoided entirely for people with autoimmune diseases. Coffee can be an immune stimulant and its ingestion can lead to a flare, so it should also be avoided.

THE ANTI-INFLAMMATORY DIET AT A GLANCE

Here is a quick cheat sheet for foods to enjoy and foods to avoid, to help you live well with lupus.

FOODS THAT FIGHT INFLAMMATION

- Meat and poultry, including organ meats: choose antibiotic-free, hormone-free, organic, and grass-fed or pasture-raised, if possible

- Fatty fish high in omega-3s: wild salmon, sardines, mussels, rainbow trout, Atlantic mackerel

- All vegetables, except nightshades (see the list below)

- All fruits, in moderation (no more than two servings per day)

- Sweet potatoes and other tubers

- Fresh and dried herbs

- Coconut products (oil, butter, sugar, meat, etc.)

- Oils and fats: avocado oil, coconut oil, olive oil

- Fermented foods: coconut milk yogurt, kombucha, nondairy kefir, sauer-kraut, white kimchi

- Sweeteners: honey, real maple syrup

- Bone broth (*must* be made from real bones; the canned broth at stores does not contain the important minerals or collagen found in real bone broth and is loaded with sodium)

- Green, black, and most herbal teas

- Vinegar

FOODS THAT WORSEN INFLAMMATION

- All grains, including wheat, barley, rye, rice, quinoa, and oats

- Eggs

- Dairy

- Beans and legumes

- Tofu

- Sugar

- Non-nutritive sweeteners (Splenda, stevia, Equal, aspartame, etc.)

- Food additives and thickeners (emulsifiers, artificial colors and flavors, etc.)

- All fats except those listed above

- Nuts and seeds

- Chocolate

- Alcohol

- Coffee

Tips to Make Home Cooking Easier

Set yourself up for success in cooking and preparing food; it can only make sticking with your diet easier. When you are tired or in pain, you probably don't want to do much prep, so it's important to have everything you need on hand to make cooking as simple as possible. Here are some great tips for setting up your kitchen to make cooking and eating with lupus easier.

LUPUS-FRIENDLY KITCHEN STAPLES

To make the recipes in this book as simple to prepare as possible, without having to run to the store all the time, there are certain pantry items you should have on hand. I've chosen these based on what you'll use most often for preparing the dishes in this book.

MUST-HAVE PANTRY STAPLES:

- Avocado oil
- Canned plain pumpkin purée
- Coconut flour
- Coconut milk, canned
- Coconut oil
- Dried fruit (such as figs, blueberries, and cranberries)
- Extra-virgin olive oil
- Honey (local if possible)
- Unflavored gelatin
- Unsweetened shredded coconut

HERBS AND SPICES:

- Black pepper
- Dried basil
- Dried oregano

- Garlic powder

- Ground cinnamon

- Ground ginger

- Ground turmeric

- Onion powder

- Sea salt

REFRIGERATOR STAPLES:

- Cauliflower

- Fresh garlic

- Fresh herbs

- Green leafy vegetables (such as collard greens, kale, and lettuce)

- Lemons and limes

- Onions

- Summer or winter squash (depending on the season)

- Sweet potatoes

FREEZER STAPLES:

- Frozen bananas

- Frozen mixed berries

- Organic, grass-fed ground beef

- Organic, pasture-raised, hormone-free, and antibiotic-free chicken

- Wild-caught frozen fish

KITCHEN EQUIPMENT

If you want to make cooking easy, have the right equipment. This can be particularly helpful during flares. You'll need a basic cookware set of saucepan, stockpot, and large skillet, plus a baking sheet and a ceramic baking dish.

Nonstick cookware can be toxic and may trigger more inflammation, so stick with stainless steel or cast iron. Here is a list of other utensils and appliances that will be helpful to have on hand.

ESSENTIAL

- Basic microwave oven
- Bendable cutting boards
- Chef's knife and paring knife
- Electric can opener
- Electric jar opener
- Food processor
- Garlic press
- Glass storage containers
- High-powered blender
- Meat thermometer
- Toaster oven

NICE TO HAVE

- Immersion blender
- Mandoline slicer
- Multi-chopper
- Pineapple slicer
- Slow cooker with liners for easy cleanup
- Spiral vegetable slicer

STICK-WITH-IT TIPS

One of the greatest challenges of any diet is to stick with it. But for best results, you must strictly follow the AIP or inflammation will return. The recipes in this book are simple and taste great, which should make the diet easy to stick to. That's my part. But you have a part to play as well. Make it easy for yourself with these tips.

Change your mind-set. This is a diet for your health, so focus on why you want to be healthy. When you want to cheat, go back to your "why."

Ask for support. Explain to your family and friends how this way of eating will help you achieve better health. Ask for their support in sticking to the plan.

Get professional help. Sometimes we need fresh ideas or someone to listen to us. A registered dietitian or counselor can help you with these aspects of sticking with the plan.

Make it easy. Buy precut, prewashed vegetables. Use frozen vegetables, if necessary.

Always have a few items on hand that don't require cooking. This way, when you are too tired to cook, you can still eat right.

Consider a meal-delivery service when you are in a flare. There are so many services these days that will deliver appropriate meals to your home. They can ease the burden of cooking.

COOKING FOR THE REST OF YOUR FAMILY

When others in your home don't have lupus, it can be challenging for them to understand your diet restrictions. Consider having them read this book or other information on the AIP diet. Explain the anti-inflammatory benefits of this way of eating and how it will help improve your pain and fatigue. Ask for their support.

Be specific about the type of support you need. Do you want them to help you grocery shop? Prepare meals? Or do you just want them not to keep prohibited foods in the house? The more specific you can be, the more likely they will know what type of support you need and be able to give it.

If you have children or other people who don't need to follow such a strict diet, you may feel you need to cook two different meals. But this is not the case. Everyone can eat meat and vegetables, and you can just add a grain or a starch to their meal if that makes it feel more complete for them.

EATING OUT WITH LUPUS

Eating out can be a major challenge when following the AIP. It can be really exhausting to worry all the time about what ingredients are in a dish that can lead to a flare. But eating out is part of everyone's social life. The key is to arrive prepared, by doing your research ahead of time. Many restaurants now have menus online, and you can check out ingredients before you go. Once you arrive, be sure to ask plenty of questions if you are not sure what might be included in a particular dish. Here are a few recommendations based on different types of foods.

CUISINE	CHOOSE	AVOID
American	Protein with a side of vegetables; salads with chicken, fish, or steak	Baked potatoes, bread, French fries, pasta, rice
Asian	Chicken, fish, vegetables	Breaded/fried protein, rice, sauces with sugar such as orange sauce or teriyaki, soy sauce (contains gluten, but many places do offer gluten-free soy sauce)
Italian	Fish or chicken with a side of vegetables	Pasta and tomato sauce
Mexican	Carne asada, ceviche (no tomatoes), fajitas (no peppers), guacamole (if it doesn't have tomatoes), seafood dishes, shrimp	Beans, cheese, chile peppers, peppers, tomatoes, tortillas, tortilla chips

About the Recipes

The recipes in this book were developed with both flavor and nutrition in mind—you'll never feel like you're missing out on old favorites. They also have labels that match different aspects of your lupus journey and will help you identify specific recipes that might match your particular concerns. Any of these recipes can work for someone with lupus, but it is such a varied disease and affects people so differently that sometimes you just need a specific food for a specific problem. Here are the labels you will find.

Flare Soother: These anti-inflammatory recipes are most recommended during a flare. They are full of foods that fight inflammation.

Fatigue-Friendly: These are the easiest recipes possible, for when you are just too tired to cook.

Kidney Support: Lupus attacks the kidneys in some people. If you have kidney damage, it is important to protect the kidneys by avoiding certain types of foods. Look for these recipes if this is the case.

Cardio Care: These recipes are helpful for people with heart problems, such as high cholesterol or high blood pressure.

Bone Booster: These recipes are high in calcium, vitamin D, and other minerals to help support bone health.

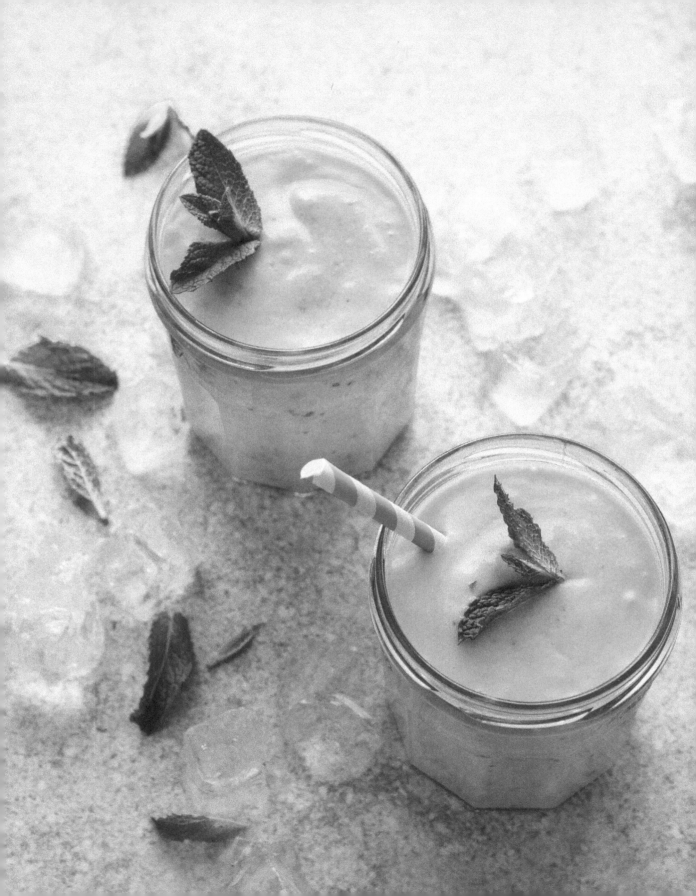

2 Smoothies and Breakfasts

CANTALOUPE MINT SMOOTHIE

| FLARE SOOTHER | FATIGUE-FRIENDLY | CARDIO CARE | BONE BOOSTER |

Cantaloupe is high in beta-carotene, making the juicy summer treat a great immune booster. This smoothie will keep well in the refrigerator, which is why the recipe serves two. Enjoy it as a snack or part of a quick breakfast on a hot day. It is particularly refreshing in the summer.

SERVES 2

Prep time: 5 minutes

2 cups chopped cantaloupe

4 or 5 fresh mint leaves

1 (10.5-ounce) can coconut milk

Handful of ice

In a blender, combine all the ingredients. Process until smooth.

SUBSTITUTION TIP: Try this smoothie with any other melon you enjoy. Watermelon, muskmelon, and honeydew all taste great as smoothies.

Per serving: Calories 395; Total fat 36g; Saturated fat 32g; Cholesterol 0mg; Carbs 21g; Fiber 5g; Protein 5g; Sodium 47mg

CARROT PEAR COCONUT SMOOTHIE

FLARE SOOTHER | FATIGUE-FRIENDLY | CARDIO CARE | BONE BOOSTER

This bright smoothie is the perfect start to your day. Naturally sweet from the combination of carrots, pear, and coconut, this smoothie is great for cleansing the body. Much of a carrot's nutrients are concentrated in and near its skin, which is why it's best to leave the carrot unpeeled when blending. Simply scrub it well before chopping.

SERVES 1

Prep time: 5 minutes

1 carrot, chopped

½ pear, cored and roughly chopped

¾ cup coconut milk

1 cup mixed greens (kale, spinach, collards)

Handful of ice

In a blender, combine all the ingredients. Blend until smooth.

INGREDIENT TIP: Conventionally grown pears receive many applications of pesticides throughout the growing season, earning them the not-so-great distinction of being one of the most toxic fruits. For this reason, try to buy organic pears.

Per serving: Calories 512; Total fat 43g; Saturated fat 38g; Cholesterol 0mg; Carbs 34g; Fiber 9g; Protein 7g; Sodium 99mg

RASPBERRY LIME SMOOTHIE

FLARE SOOTHER | FATIGUE-FRIENDLY | CARDIO CARE | BONE BOOSTER

Not much tastes more like summer than fresh berries. Make this when raspberries are in season, or use frozen raspberries to enjoy the flavor year round. If you use fresh berries, add a handful of ice to the blender.

SERVES 1

Prep time: 5 minutes

1 cup frozen raspberries

1 cup baby spinach

Juice of 1 lime

¾ cup coconut milk

1 teaspoon honey

In a blender, combine all the ingredients. Process until smooth.

SUBSTITUTION TIP: No lime? For another great flavor combination, use fresh lemon.

Per serving: Calories 513; Total fat 43g; Saturated fat 38g; Cholesterol 0mg; Carbs 35g; Fiber 9g; Protein 7g; Sodium 52mg

SWEET AVOCADO AND GREENS SMOOTHIE

FLARE SOOTHER | FATIGUE-FRIENDLY | CARDIO CARE | BONE BOOSTER

Avocados are a wonderful source of monounsaturated fatty acids, vitamin E, and many B vitamins. Adding one to your smoothie in the morning is a great way to start your day with heart-healthy fats. Get two servings of vegetables and one serving of fruit first thing in the morning with this easy drink, and you will be on your way to a great day.

SERVES 1

Prep time: 5 minutes

½ avocado, pitted and peeled

1 cup spinach or kale

½ apple, cored and roughly chopped

¾ cup coconut milk

Handful of ice

In a blender, combine the avocado, spinach, apple, and coconut milk. Add the ice and process until smooth.

INGREDIENT TIP: When you are using only half an avocado, be sure to leave the pit in the unused half until you are ready to use it. Refrigerate in an airtight container.

Per serving: Calories 623; Total fat 57g; Saturated fat 40g; Cholesterol 0mg; Carbs 34g; Fiber 13g; Protein 7g; Sodium 59mg

MATCHA AND BERRY SMOOTHIE BOWL

| FLARE SOOTHER | FATIGUE-FRIENDLY | CARDIO CARE | BONE BOOSTER |

Smoothie bowls are a fun way to eat a smoothie with some extras. Create a base using coconut, berries, greens, and matcha, and top with additional berries and coconut flakes for a delicious breakfast that is ready in minutes. Typically a little thicker than a traditional smoothie, this is a smoothie you eat with a spoon, adding a berry or coconut flake to each bite for added texture and popping flavor.

SERVES 2

Prep time: 5 minutes

¼ cup unsweetened shredded coconut

2 cups mixed berries (raspberries, strawberries, blueberries), divided

2 cups mixed greens (spinach, kale)

1 cup full-fat coconut milk

1 tablespoon matcha powder

Handful of ice

2 tablespoons toasted coconut flakes

1. In a blender, combine the coconut, 1½ cups of the berries, the greens, coconut milk, matcha powder, and a handful of ice, and process until smooth. Pour into two bowls.

2. Top each bowl with ¼ cup of berries and 1 tablespoon of coconut flakes.

INGREDIENT TIP: Matcha is a green-tea powder that is loaded with more antioxidants than the steeped version of green tea. Because you are consuming the entire leaf of the tea instead of water steeped in the tea leaves, matcha is a better source of nutrients than green tea. Look for it at health food stores and Asian supermarkets.

Per serving: Calories 454; Total fat 41g; Saturated fat 36g; Cholesterol 0mg; Carbs 23g; Fiber 10g; Protein 6g; Sodium 51mg

BLUEBERRY BREAKFAST SMOOTHIE BOWL

FLARE SOOTHER | FATIGUE-FRIENDLY | CARDIO CARE | BONE BOOSTER

Blueberries are loaded with antioxidants, vitamin C, and fiber, making them a super way to start your morning. This luscious smoothie bowl is creamy with coconut milk and kissed with cinnamon, which helps promote stable blood sugar. The banana provides a great texture, and the extra berries and banana pieces on top make this bowl so much more fun to eat than a simple smoothie.

SERVES 2

Prep time: 5 minutes

1 cup frozen
blueberries, divided

1 banana, sliced, divided

2 cups baby spinach

¾ cup coconut milk

1 teaspoon ground cinnamon

Handful of ice

1. In a blender, combine ¾ cup of the blueberries, ¾ of the banana slices, the spinach, coconut milk, cinnamon, and ice. Process until smooth.

2. Pour into two bowls. Top with the reserved blueberries and banana slices.

SUBSTITUTION TIP: Substitute any leafy green for the spinach. Collard greens, kale, turnip greens, mustard greens, and even radish greens can all be nutrient-dense additions to smoothies and smoothie bowls.

Per serving: Calories 311; Total fat 22g; Saturated fat 19g; Cholesterol 0mg; Carbs 31g; Fiber 7g; Protein 4g; Sodium 38mg

BREAKFAST SALAD BOWL

FLARE SOOTHER │ FATIGUE-FRIENDLY │ BONE BOOSTER

Salad for breakfast is a great idea. Start your morning off with this fresh salad loaded with heart-healthy fat and plenty of flavor. Oranges provide sweetness and are the backbone of the dressing. A slice of prosciutto ties the whole thing together and makes this simple dish all the more satisfying.

SERVES 1

Prep time: 5 minutes

2 cups mixed salad greens

1 tablespoon extra-virgin olive oil

1 small mandarin orange, peeled and segmented

Pinch sea salt

Freshly ground black pepper

½ avocado, sliced

1 slice prosciutto

1. In a medium bowl, toss the salad greens and olive oil. Squeeze the juice from 2 or 3 of the orange segments over the greens and stir to combine. Season with salt and pepper and mix in the remaining orange segments.

2. Serve the salad topped with the avocado and prosciutto.

COOKING TIP: Make the salad the night before and let it marinate in the dressing overnight. In the morning, cut the avocado and add it plus the prosciutto for a quick meal.

Per serving: Calories 410; Total fat 32g; Saturated fat 5g; Cholesterol 25mg; Carbs 25g; Fiber 10g; Protein 14g; Sodium 932mg

BREAKFAST GREEN SOUP

FLARE SOOTHER | FATIGUE-FRIENDLY | CARDIO CARE | BONE BOOSTER

Soup for breakfast may not be one of the first things that come to mind when you are changing your diet, but this is a delicious way to start your day. Loaded with kale, this soup is rich in beta-carotene, vitamin C, collagen, and anti-inflammatory amino acids such as glutamine, which help support the immune system. Pour it in a cup and drink it down for a quick and nutritious breakfast.

SERVES 2

Prep time: 5 minutes

Cook time: 10 minutes

1 tablespoon extra-virgin olive oil

1 small onion, chopped

2 cups Chicken Bone Broth (page 151)

1 tablespoon unflavored gelatin

6 cups chopped kale

Juice of ½ lime

Sea salt

Freshly ground black pepper

1. In a medium pan, heat the olive oil over medium-high heat. Add the onion and cook for 3 to 5 minutes until translucent.

2. Add the chicken broth and gelatin, stirring well to dissolve the gelatin. Add the kale and bring to a simmer. Reduce the heat and cook for 3 to 5 minutes until the kale wilts.

3. Using an immersion blender or in a regular blender, purée the soup. Add the lime juice and season with salt and pepper.

SUBSTITUTION TIP: Use chard or spinach in place of kale.

Per serving: Calories 200; Total fat 7g; Saturated fat 1g; Cholesterol 0mg; Carbs 27g; Fiber 4g; Protein 11g; Sodium 260mg

BUTTERNUT SQUASH PORRIDGE

| FLARE SOOTHER | FATIGUE-FRIENDLY | KIDNEY SUPPORT | CARDIO CARE | BONE BOOSTER |

While oats and other grain-based porridges are out, that doesn't mean you can't still enjoy a bowl of warm breakfast porridge. This squash porridge is rich and creamy— a great source of complex carbohydrates and beta-carotene.

SERVES 2

Prep time: 10 minutes

Cook time: 55 minutes

1 butternut squash, halved and seeded

1 cup Chicken Bone Broth (page 151)

½ cup coconut milk

1 teaspoon pure maple syrup

2 teaspoons ground cinnamon

Pinch sea salt

1. Preheat the oven to 350°F.

2. In a baking dish, place the squash, cut-side down. Add ¼ cup of water and bake for 45 to 50 minutes until the squash is tender when a fork is inserted.

3. Scoop the flesh out of the squash and transfer to a medium pot. Using a potato masher, mash the flesh until smooth. Add the broth, coconut milk, maple syrup, and cinnamon to the pot. Season with salt. Stir well and heat over medium heat.

4. Once it's simmering, turn off the heat and serve. Drizzle with a little additional coconut milk and sprinkle with more cinnamon, if desired.

COOKING TIP: Bake the squash and mash it the night before, then mix all the remaining ingredients in the morning for a quick breakfast. Or make it the night before and reheat the porridge in the morning. The overnight rest intensifies the flavors.

Per serving: Calories 315; Total fat 15g; Saturated fat 13g; Cholesterol 0mg; Carbs 49g; Fiber 10g; Protein 6g; Sodium 146mg

FRUITY GRANOLA

| FLARE SOOTHER | FATIGUE-FRIENDLY | KIDNEY SUPPORT | CARDIO CARE | BONE BOOSTER |

It can be hard to give up breakfast cereals and granola when you're on a grain-free diet. With this super simple granola, you can still enjoy the crunch and flavor of granola without risking a flare. Dried fruits and coconut flakes stand in for the grains. Be sure to check the labels to ensure that no inflammatory oils or additives are included in the dried figs and blueberries.

SERVES 6

Prep time: 5 minutes

Cook time: 12 minutes

2 cups unsweetened coconut flakes

1 cup sliced dried figs

1 cup dried blueberries

2 tablespoons coconut oil, melted

1 teaspoon ground cinnamon

1 teaspoon pure maple syrup

¼ teaspoon sea salt

1. Preheat the oven to 350°F. Line a baking sheet with parchment paper.

2. In a medium bowl, toss the coconut flakes, figs, blueberries, coconut oil, cinnamon, maple syrup, and salt. Spread mixture onto baking sheet.

3. Bake for 12 minutes, flipping once about halfway through.

4. Let cool to room temperature, then store in an airtight container for up to 1 week in the refrigerator.

SUBSTITUTION TIP: Use other dried fruits, such as apples, raisins, dates, currants, cherries, or bananas, in place of the figs and blueberries.

Per serving: Calories 282; Total fat 18g; Saturated fat 16g; Cholesterol 0mg; Carbs 33g; Fiber 7g; Protein 3g; Sodium 88mg

COCONUT BANANA BREAKFAST COOKIES

FLARE SOOTHER | FATIGUE-FRIENDLY | CARDIO CARE

On busy mornings, these sweet breakfast cookies are a life saver. Made using just three ingredients, they are as simple as can be and taste great, too. Make a batch of these on Sunday and grab them all week for a quick breakfast on the go.

MAKES 10 COOKIES (2 COOKIES PER SERVING)

Prep time: 5 minutes

Cook time: 25 minutes

Nonstick cooking spray

2 bananas, peeled

1½ cups unsweetened shredded coconut

½ cup dried blueberries

1. Preheat the oven to 350°F. Lightly spray a baking sheet with nonstick cooking spray.

2. In a food processor, pulse the bananas and coconut until well combined. Stir in the blueberries.

3. Shape the mixture into 10 discs and arrange on the prepared sheet. Bake for 25 minutes until golden brown. Cool on the baking sheet for 10 minutes before removing with a spatula.

4. Store the cookies in an airtight container in the refrigerator for up to 5 days.

SUBSTITUTION TIP: You can substitute dried currants, cherries, and raisins for the blueberries here. Just be sure no sugar or other additives were used in their processing.

Per serving: Calories 186; Total fat 13g; Saturated fat 11g; Cholesterol 0mg; Carbs 19g; Fiber 5g; Protein 2g; Sodium 8mg

GRAIN-FREE PUMPKIN PANCAKES

FLARE SOOTHER | FATIGUE-FRIENDLY | CARDIO CARE

Although you can't eat grain pancakes, these simple four-ingredient cakes can take their place and fill it well. Coconut flour helps bind the ingredients, and both the banana and pumpkin add a light sweetness. Be sure to cook the pancakes on medium-low heat to allow them to set without burning; they take a little longer than a traditional pancake.

SERVES 2

Prep time: 5 minutes

2 ripe bananas

½ cup plain pumpkin purée

¼ cup coconut flour

1 teaspoon ground cinnamon

2 tablespoons coconut oil

Pure maple syrup or honey, for serving

1. In a food processor, combine the bananas, pumpkin, coconut flour, and cinnamon and process until smooth. If necessary, add up to 2 tablespoons of water to create a smooth consistency.

2. In a large skillet, heat the coconut oil over medium-low heat.

3. Add a large spoonful of batter to the skillet and spread so that it is about ½ inch thick. Cook for 3 to 4 minutes until browned and set, then flip and cook for 3 to 4 minutes more. Repeat with the remaining batter.

4. Serve topped with pure maple syrup or honey.

COOKING TIP: These pancakes do not firm up as quickly as traditional wheat and egg–based pancakes, so be sure to take it slow when cooking. Use a metal spatula when flipping for the best results.

Per serving: Calories 366; Total fat 17g; Saturated fat 14g; Cholesterol 0mg; Carbs 53g; Fiber 18g; Protein 6g; Sodium 4mg

SQUASH SCRAMBLE SKILLET

FLARE SOOTHER | FATIGUE-FRIENDLY | CARDIO CARE | BONE BOOSTER

The varieties of hard winter squash to try these days are amazing. Because delicata squash is a thin-skinned variety, it doesn't need to be peeled, making the prep work minimal. With a medley of vegetables, this lovely skillet is colorful and tasty. This scramble keeps well in the refrigerator, so you can enjoy it throughout the week for breakfast.

SERVES 4

Prep time: 5 minutes

Cook time: 30 minutes

2 tablespoons coconut oil

1 small delicata squash, seeded and chopped

1 small onion, chopped

3 garlic cloves, minced

2 cups chopped cauliflower florets

1 cup sliced mushrooms

4 cups chopped Swiss chard

Sea salt

1. In a large skillet, heat the coconut oil over medium-high heat. Add the squash and cook, stirring regularly, for about 15 minutes until just fork tender.

2. Add the onion and cook for 2 to 3 minutes more until browned. Add the garlic and stir until fragrant, about 30 seconds. Add the cauliflower and mushrooms and cook for 5 to 7 minutes until softened.

3. Add the chard, a handful at a time, stirring until it wilts before adding more. Season with salt and serve.

SUBSTITUTION TIP: To avoid the chopping and peeling altogether, substitute about 2 cups of ready-cut fresh butternut squash or another type of winter squash available at your local store.

Per serving: Calories 139; Total fat 7g; Saturated fat 6g; Cholesterol 0mg; Carbs 19g; Fiber 5g; Protein 4g; Sodium 137mg

SWEET POTATO, KALE, AND MUSHROOM SCRAMBLE

FLARE SOOTHER | **CARDIO CARE** | **BONE BOOSTER**

This veggie scramble is so easy, and you can customize it to your taste. Serve it on its own or pair it with the Chicken Breakfast Sausage (page 39). Be sure to chop the sweet potatoes finely so that they cook quickly. Make the whole batch and enjoy this throughout the week; it reheats well and makes for a quick breakfast on a busy morning.

SERVES 4

Prep time: 5 minutes

Cook time: 25 minutes

1 tablespoon coconut oil

1 small onion, chopped

2 garlic cloves, minced

2 sweet potatoes, finely chopped

4 cups chopped kale

2½ cups sliced mushrooms

Sea salt

1. In a large skillet, heat the coconut oil over medium heat. Sauté the onion and garlic for 3 to 5 minutes, stirring regularly, until translucent.

2. Add the sweet potatoes and cook, stirring occasionally, for 10 to 15 minutes until the sweet potatoes are cooked through.

3. Add the kale and mushrooms to the skillet and toss until the kale and mushrooms are wilted. Season with salt and serve.

VARIATION TIP: For even more flavor, at the end of cooking add ¼ to ½ cup of coconut milk to the scramble and stir well.

Per serving: Calories 133; Total fat 4g; Saturated fat 3g; Cholesterol 0mg; Carbs 23g; Fiber 4g; Protein 4g; Sodium 126mg

SWEET POTATO AND BACON HASH

FLARE SOOTHER | CARDIO CARE | BONE BOOSTER

Sweet potatoes are part of several breakfasts here because they are a perfect fuel in the morning. Loaded with vitamins A and C and antioxidants, they are a nutrient-dense tuber that just tastes great. Here, they are paired with bacon and spinach for a sweet and salty scramble you will enjoy again and again.

SERVES 4

Prep time: 5 minutes

Cook time: 25 minutes

4 bacon slices, chopped

2 tablespoons extra-virgin olive oil

1 small onion, chopped

2 medium sweet potatoes, chopped into ¼-inch pieces

4 cups finely chopped spinach

2 tablespoons chopped parsley

¼ teaspoon sea salt

1. In a large skillet over medium heat, cook the bacon for 5 to 7 minutes until crispy. Transfer to a plate lined with paper towels. Remove the bacon grease from the pan.

2. Heat the olive oil in the same skillet and cook the onion for 3 to 5 minutes until just starting to soften. Add the sweet potatoes and cook for 12 to 15 minutes until the sweet potatoes are browned and tender.

3. Stir in the spinach and cook, stirring, until the spinach wilts. Add the parsley and cooked bacon and stir well. Season with salt and serve.

INGREDIENT TIP: Try using different types of sweet potato when making scrambles such as this, to switch things up a bit. While orange-flesh sweet potatoes are most commonly available, white- and even purple-flesh varieties are really fun to experiment with for a slightly different flavor.

Per serving: Calories 233; Total fat 15g; Saturated fat 4g; Cholesterol 21mg; Carbs 16g; Fiber 3g; Protein 9g; Sodium 617mg

CHICKEN BREAKFAST SAUSAGE

FLARE SOOTHER	FATIGUE-FRIENDLY	KIDNEY SUPPORT	CARDIO CARE	BONE BOOSTER

Most store-bought breakfast sausages are filled with a variety of off-limit additives, fillers, and spices. This simple recipe is nearly as easy as buying premade, and completely complies with the autoimmune diet to help support your body's healing.

SERVES 4

Prep time: 5 minutes

Cook time: 10 minutes

1 pound ground chicken

1 tablespoon pure maple syrup

½ teaspoon sea salt

1 teaspoon dried sage

1 teaspoon garlic powder

1 tablespoon coconut oil

1. In a large mixing bowl, combine the chicken, maple syrup, salt, sage, and garlic powder. Mix well.

2. Shape the mixture into four patties.

3. In a large skillet, heat the coconut oil over medium-high heat. Place the patties in the skillet and cook for 3 to 4 minutes for each side until browned and cooked through.

SUBSTITUTION TIP: You can substitute pork if you prefer it or simply want a change of pace. Just use an equal amount of ground pork instead of the chicken.

Per serving: Calories 205; Total fat 13g; Saturated fat 6g; Cholesterol 96mg; Carbs 4g; Fiber 0g; Protein 20g; Sodium 302mg

CHICKEN BREAKFAST SKILLET

FLARE SOOTHER | CARDIO CARE | BONE BOOSTER

This is just one fun way to play around with the Chicken Breakfast Sausage (page 39). If you are making the sausage from scratch, don't shape it into patties but instead just fry it in a pan and crumble it. This reheats well so make a full batch and heat it up for breakfast throughout the week.

SERVES 4

Prep time: 5 minutes

Cook time: 20 minutes

1 tablespoon coconut oil

1 recipe uncooked Chicken Breakfast Sausage (page 39) or 1 pound ground chicken

2 cups chopped carrots

2 cups peeled and chopped butternut squash

½ cup water

1 tablespoon Chimichurri Sauce (page 163)

3 cups baby arugula

Sea salt

1. In a large skillet, heat the coconut oil over medium heat. Brown the breakfast sausage over medium heat, stirring to break up the chunks as it cooks. Remove from the skillet with a slotted spoon, so the oil stays in the pan, and set aside.

2. Add the carrots, squash, and water to the skillet. Cover and cook for 5 to 6 minutes until just fork tender. Remove the lid and continue to cook for 4 or 5 more minutes until all the liquid evaporates and the squash and carrots brown slightly.

3. Stir in the chimichurri sauce and return the sausage to the skillet. Mix well. Add the arugula and stir until just wilted. Season with salt and serve.

INGREDIENT TIP: Chimichurri is a great sauce to have on hand for seasoning a variety of dishes. Freeze it in ice-cube trays so you have perfectly portioned amounts on hand for easy use.

Per serving: Calories 247; Total fat 13g; Saturated fat 6g; Cholesterol 96mg; Carbs 14g; Fiber 3g; Protein 21g; Sodium 151mg

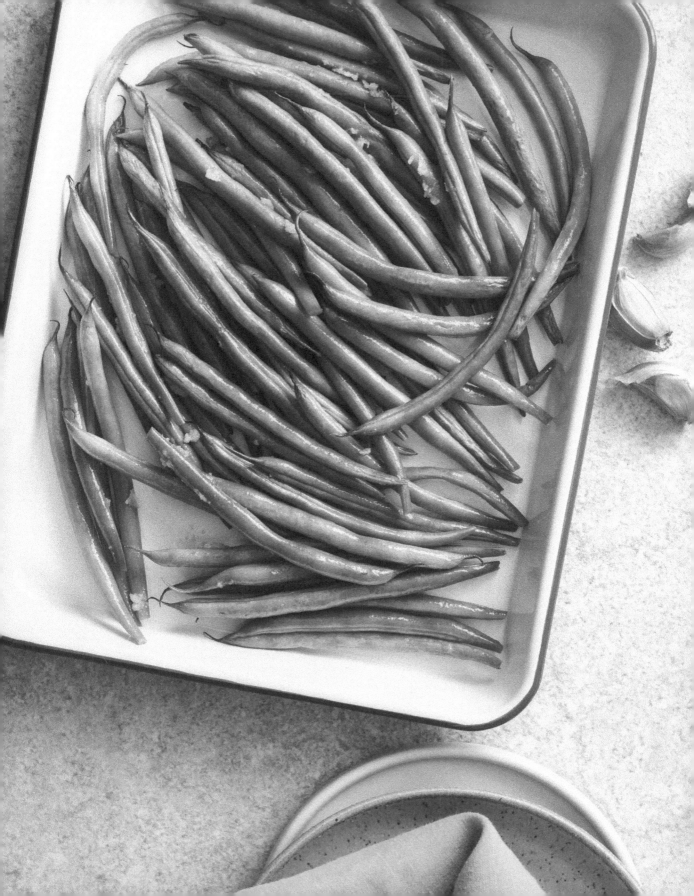

3 Snacks and Sides

CINNAMON APPLE CHIPS

If you have an apple corer, you can make circular chips, but if not, don't let that stop you from making this simple recipe. Half-circle chips are just as tasty and require no special equipment. Be sure to leave the skin on, as it is loaded with fiber. If you have a mandoline, use it for this recipe. Aim for slices between ⅛ inch and ¼ inch thick.

SERVES 4

Prep time: 5 minutes

Cook time: 2 to 3 hours

Nonstick olive oil cooking spray

4 apples, cored and thinly sliced

1 teaspoon ground cinnamon

1. Preheat the oven to 200°F. Lightly spray two baking sheets with nonstick cooking spray.

2. In a medium bowl, toss the apples with the cinnamon. Arrange the apples in a single layer on the prepared baking sheets.

3. Bake for 2 to 3 hours until the apples are dry but still soft and pliable. Let cool completely; they will crisp up as they cool.

4. Transfer to an airtight container and store at room temperature for up to 3 days or in the refrigerator for several weeks.

INGREDIENT TIP: Use your favorite type of apple for this recipe, as its flavor will really come through in the finished chips. Granny Smith and Fuji apples are my favorites for making chips.

Per serving: Calories 117; Total fat 0g; Saturated fat 0g; Cholesterol 0mg; Carbs 31g; Fiber 6g; Protein 1g; Sodium 2mg

COLLARD GREENS CHIPS

FLARE SOOTHER	FATIGUE-FRIENDLY	CARDIO CARE	BONE BOOSTER

No one is ever saying you should eat more chips, unless they are these amazingly healthy and delicious collards. Kale chips have been a popular health food for years, but these similar chips made from collard greens are just as easy to make and have even more bite. The bitter green pairs well with many different flavors, making them just as versatile and easy as kale chips. You can make them even easier by just using olive oil, salt, and collards. Experiment with what you like and keep making more.

SERVES 2

Prep time: 5 minutes

Cook time: 20 minutes

3 garlic cloves, finely minced

2 tablespoons extra-virgin olive oil

1 teaspoon apple cider vinegar

1 teaspoon coconut aminos

1 teaspoon honey

Sea salt

1 pound collard greens, thick stems removed, leaves chopped

1. Preheat the oven to 300°F. Line two baking sheets with parchment paper.

2. In a large bowl, whisk together the garlic, olive oil, vinegar, coconut aminos, and honey. Season with salt. Stir in the collard greens, mixing well to ensure all the pieces are coated.

3. On the prepared baking sheets, spread the collard greens in a single layer. Bake for 18 to 20 minutes. After 10 minutes of cooking, begin checking on the chips every few minutes. As some chips finish cooking and become crisp, transfer them to another plate. Continue until all are done. Let the chips cool before serving.

4. Store in an airtight container for up to 3 days.

INGREDIENT TIP: Coconut aminos, one of the main flavor components here, is a salty sauce that is a great substitute for soy sauce. Made from the fermented sap of coconut blossom nectar, it is slightly sweet and significantly less salty than soy sauce. Find it at health food stores, Caribbean markets, or online.

Per serving: Calories 203; Total fat 16g; Saturated fat 2g; Cholesterol 0mg; Carbs 17g; Fiber 8g; Protein 5g; Sodium 158mg

PLANTAIN WRAPS

FLARE SOOTHER | FATIGUE-FRIENDLY | BONE BOOSTER

Just because you can't eat grains doesn't mean you have to give up sandwiches. These simple and nutritious wraps are perfect for tuna or chicken salad, pulled pork, any of the breakfast scrambles or side dishes in this book—or anything else you want in a wrap. You can also break them into pieces and use with any of the salsa or dips in chapter 9. They're a bit spongy rather than crispy but will still be delicious as a chip substitute. While they do keep for a couple of days when refrigerated, they are best right out of the oven.

SERVES 4

Prep time: 5 minutes

Cook time: 25 minutes

2 cups chopped green plantains

¼ cup coconut oil

½ teaspoon sea salt

½ cup water

1. Preheat the oven to 375°F. Line a baking sheet with parchment paper.

2. In a blender, combine the plantains, coconut oil, salt, and water. Process until smooth.

3. Transfer to the prepared baking sheet and spread into a thin, even layer across the sheet.

4. Bake for 25 minutes until set and browned. Cut into four pieces and use as wraps for sandwiches, or break into chips.

INGREDIENT TIP: It is important to choose green plantains for this recipe, as you want the batter to be more starchy than sweet. While many recipes start by boiling them, I find that they work well just as they are. To remove the green plantain from its skin, you will need to slit the skin with a kitchen knife and firmly peel it from the flesh.

Per serving: Calories 208; Total fat 14g; Saturated fat 12g; Cholesterol 0mg; Carbs 24g; Fiber 2g; Protein 1g; Sodium 237mg

COCONUT MILK YOGURT

Coconut milk makes great yogurt, and it is about as simple as can be to make. This easy ferment requires no heating and comes out great every time. Ferment the yogurt for 24 hours or even up to 48 hours for a super tangy flavor.

**MAKES 24 OUNCES
(6 OUNCES PER SERVING)**

Prep time: 5 minutes

Fermentation time: 24 hours

2 (14-ounce) cans full-fat coconut milk

2 probiotic capsules

1. Pour the coconut milk into a quart jar.

2. Open the probiotic capsules and empty their contents into the coconut milk. Discard the capsules. Stir well.

3. Cover with cheesecloth, secure with a rubber band, and place in a room temperature location for 24 hours until tangy and thickened slightly.

4. Screw on a tight-fitting lid and refrigerate for 5 to 7 days.

VARIATION TIP: Depending on the type of coconut milk and probiotics you use, the results will vary in thickness. If you want a thicker yogurt, stir a teaspoon of gelatin into the finished yogurt and store in the refrigerator to thicken.

Per serving: Calories 228; Total fat 24g; Saturated fat 21g; Cholesterol 0mg; Carbs 6g; Fiber 2g; Protein 2g; Sodium 15mg

FERMENTED CARROT STICKS

FATIGUE-FRIENDLY | KIDNEY SUPPORT

Fermented carrots are a great snack, and the flavor can range from lightly pickled to full-on soured, depending on how long you let them ferment. I prefer to stop the fermentation process after a few days, but you can certainly let them go longer if you want more of a pickled taste. Pair these with Cauli-Ranch Dip (page 162) for a delightful vegetable-based snack. Pickling salt is used in canning and pickling. Like table salt, it's sodium chloride, but unlike table salt, it does not contain iodine and anticaking additives, which can cause unappealing cloudiness in the finished pickles.

SERVES 2

Prep time: 5 minutes
Fermentation time: 2 to 7 days

1 pound carrots, scrubbed and cut into sticks

3 garlic cloves, peeled and smashed

1 tablespoon fine sea salt or pickling salt

2 cups filtered water

1. Pack the carrot strips and garlic into a quart jar.

2. In a small bowl, dissolve the salt in the water. Pour the liquid over the carrots, leaving about 2 inches of space at the top of the jar. If needed, use a weight to hold the carrots down below the brine.

3. Cover the jar with a coffee filter, airlock top, or tight lid. Set in a room temperature (60°F to 70°F) location for 2 to 10 days until they reach the desired flavor and texture. The shorter the fermentation, the crisper and more lightly pickled the carrots will be; a longer fermentation time will yield a slightly more tender and sour pickle.

4. When the carrots are fermented to your liking, cover with a tight-fitting lid and transfer to the refrigerator to stop fermentation. Store in the refrigerator for up to 2 weeks.

INGREDIENT TIP: Filtered water is important for fermentation, as additives such as fluoride and chlorine in the water supply can inhibit fermentation. Use filtered tap water, or at the very least, let your tap water stand overnight before using it, to allow some of the chlorine to dissipate.

Per serving: Calories 100; Total fat 0g; Saturated fat 0g; Cholesterol 0mg; Carbs 24g; Fiber 6g; Protein 2g; Sodium 738mg

FERMENTED CAULIFLOWER PICKLES

FATIGUE-FRIENDLY | **KIDNEY SUPPORT**

Cauliflower is one of the easiest pickles to make. Its firm texture holds up well during the fermentation process, and it is loaded with nutrients when it's ready to eat. Cauliflower already contains antioxidant, anticancer, and antibiotic characteristics, but the fermentation process ensures you get your probiotics, too. This simple pickle uses just garlic, salt, and a sprig of thyme for flavor.

SERVES 10

Prep time: 5 minutes

Fermentation time: 5 to 10 days

1 tablespoon sea salt

4 cups filtered water

1 small cauliflower head, cut into florets

3 garlic cloves, peeled and smashed

1 fresh thyme sprig

1. In a half-gallon jar or two quart jars, dissolve the salt in the water. Pack the cauliflower into the jar and add the garlic and thyme.

2. Use a small jar or other weight to hold the cauliflower below the brine. Cover the jar with a coffee filter, airlock top, or tight lid.

3. Set in a room temperature (60°F to 70°F) location for 5 to 10 days until the cauliflower reaches the desired flavor and texture. The shorter the fermentation, the crisper and more lightly pickled the cauliflower will be; a longer fermentation time will yield a slightly more tender and sour pickle.

4. When the pickles are to your liking, close the jar with a tight-fitting lid and transfer to the refrigerator to stop fermentation. Store in the refrigerator for up to 2 weeks.

COOKING TIP: This recipe will most likely not fill up an entire half-gallon jar (unless you have a really big cauliflower head) but will be more than 1 quart. Whether you divide the cauliflower and brine between two smaller jars or make it in one large jar, be sure to weight the cauliflower to hold it below the surface of the brine. If you need more brine, just mix another batch, using the same water-to-salt ratio.

Per serving: Calories 8; Total fat 0g; Saturated fat 0g; Cholesterol 0mg; Carbs 2g; Fiber 1g; Protein 1g; Sodium 124mg

SIMPLE SAUERKRAUT

FLARE SOOTHER | FATIGUE-FRIENDLY | KIDNEY SUPPORT

Sauerkraut is very simple to make at home, and with a little practice and planning you will be able to create this tasty fermented cabbage year round. Using just salt and cabbage, the process of fermentation increases vitamin C levels and makes the cruciferous vegetable even more digestible. You will need a large half-gallon jar or two smaller quart jars to make this recipe.

SERVES 2

Prep time: 15 minutes

Fermentation time: 2 to 6 weeks

1 small cabbage head (about 2 to 2½ pounds)

1½ tablespoons pickling salt

COOKING TIP: The fermentation processes used in this book are all anaerobic, meaning they take place without the presence of oxygen. For this reason, it is important to hold the produce below the brine for fermentation to take place. You may need a weight to hold the vegetables down. Use a small, clean jar or glass that fits inside the fermentation jar, or a cleaned and sanitized stone or fermentation weight to hold the cabbage down.

Per serving: Calories 142; Total fat 1g; Saturated fat 0g; Cholesterol 0mg; Carbs 33g; Fiber 14g; Protein 7g; Sodium 684mg

1. Remove and reserve two of the outer leaves from the cabbage. Remove the inner core and cut the cabbage into quarters. Using a mandoline or sharp knife, thinly slice the pieces into strips about ¼ inch thick.

2. In a large bowl, toss the cabbage with the salt and use your clean hands to evenly distribute the salt throughout the cabbage. Let rest for 10 to 15 minutes until the cabbage releases some liquid.

3. Pack the cabbage and its juices into a half-gallon jar or two quart jars. Using a clean fist or smaller jar that fits inside the large jar, pack the cabbage down firmly into the jar. Cover the cabbage shreds with the reserved cabbage leaves. If needed, use a weight to hold the cabbage below the brine. If there is not enough brine, don't worry. After 24 hours, the cabbage should release enough liquid to cover itself. Cover the jars with a lid or a clean cloth held in place with a rubber band.

4. Set the jars in a cool location, ranging from 60°F to 75°F. After a few days, you will notice bubbles rising to the top, signaling fermentation. Check the sauerkraut every couple of days, removing any scum that forms on the surface.

5. After 2 weeks, begin checking on the sauerkraut by tasting it. If the flavor is to your liking, it's ready. If not, ferment for up to 6 weeks, continuing to check and removing scum regularly.

6. When the sauerkraut is ready, remove the large cabbage leaves, cover the jar with a tight-fitting lid, and refrigerate to stop fermentation. Store in the refrigerator for up to 1 month.

TURNIP "RICE"

FATIGUE-FRIENDLY | KIDNEY SUPPORT | BONE BOOSTER

Turnips are sturdy vegetables that hold up well to being pulsed in a food processor into rice-like shards. Once riced, these grains of turnip cook up in just minutes and are ready to serve alongside your stir-fries, salads, and other main dishes.

SERVES 2

Prep time: 5 minutes

Cook time: 5 minutes

3 medium turnips, peeled and cut into 1-inch pieces

1 tablespoon extra-virgin olive oil

2 teaspoons freshly squeezed lemon juice

¼ teaspoon sea salt

1. In a food processor, pulse the turnips until they resemble rice.

2. In a large skillet, heat the olive oil over medium heat. Add the turnips and sauté for 2 to 3 minutes. Sprinkle with the lemon juice and salt and toss.

SUBSTITUTION TIP: Cauliflower and rutabaga also taste great made into rice. To do so, cut both into pieces that fit into your food processor and pulse until they resemble rice, being careful not to overprocess them into mush.

Per serving: Calories 114; Total fat 7g; Saturated fat 1g; Cholesterol 0mg; Carbs 12g; Fiber 3g; Protein 2g; Sodium 355mg

JICAMA OVEN FRIES

FATIGUE-FRIENDLY | **KIDNEY SUPPORT**

Say yes to fries when they are made with jicama. A powerful prebiotic, jicama is a root vegetable from Central America. Made up of 90 percent water (the rest being mainly fiber), it is a great stand-in for the starchy nightshade white potato. It tastes great raw, but when seasoned and cooked, it is even better. Serve these fries with Pumpkin Dip (page 161).

SERVES 2

Prep time: 5 minutes

Cook time: 55 minutes

1 medium jicama, peeled and cut into ¼-inch matchsticks

1 tablespoon extra-virgin olive oil

½ teaspoon garlic powder

½ teaspoon onion powder

½ teaspoon sea salt

1. Preheat the oven to 400°F.

2. Fill a medium pot two-thirds full with water and bring to a boil. Add the jicama and cook for 10 minutes. Drain and transfer the jicama to a medium bowl.

3. Toss the jicama with the olive oil, garlic powder, onion powder, and salt.

4. Arrange the jicama in a single layer on a baking sheet and cook for 40 to 45 minutes, flipping halfway through, until browned and crisp.

SUBSTITUTION TIP: If you don't like or can't find jicama, try rutabaga fries instead. Make the recipe the exact same way.

Per serving: Calories 190; Total fat 7g; Saturated fat 1g; Cholesterol 0mg; Carbs 30g; Fiber 16g; Protein 3g; Sodium 482mg

QUICK-ROASTED CAULIFLOWER

FLARE SOOTHER | FATIGUE-FRIENDLY | KIDNEY SUPPORT | CARDIO CARE | BONE BOOSTER

Cauliflower is a common stand-in for grain in many grain-free diets, in the form of rice, pizza crust, and more. However, this simple preparation shines on its own. Because the cauliflower is sliced, it cooks more quickly than full florets.

SERVES 4

Prep time: 5 minutes

Cook time: 20 minutes

1 cauliflower head

1 tablespoon extra-virgin olive oil

Sea salt

Juice of 1 lime

1. Preheat the oven to 425°F.

2. Break the cauliflower into florets. Using a sharp knife, cut the florets lengthwise into ½-inch slices. In a large bowl, toss the cauliflower with the olive oil and season with salt.

3. Arrange the cauliflower on a baking sheet in a single layer. Bake for 15 to 20 minutes, stirring once halfway through.

4. Squeeze the lime juice over the cauliflower and serve.

COOKING TIP: Before juicing a fresh lime, firmly roll the lime on a counter several times to soften it. This will make it much easier to extract the juice once it's cut.

Per serving: Calories 69; Total fat 4g; Saturated fat 1g; Cholesterol 0mg, Carbs 9g; Fiber 4g; Protein 3g; Sodium 82mg

SIMPLE SPAGHETTI SQUASH

Spaghetti squash is unique in that once cooked, instead of mashing apart like other hard winter squash, it separates into tiny thread-like "noodles." Serve these with any saucy dish, to help soak up the delicious flavors and to enjoy this inherently low-carb pasta alternative.

SERVES 2

Prep time: 5 minutes

Cook time: 45 minutes

1 spaghetti squash, halved lengthwise and seeded

1 tablespoon extra-virgin olive oil

Sea salt

1. Preheat the oven to 375°F.

2. Drizzle the squash with the olive oil and season lightly with salt. On a baking sheet, arrange the squash cut-side down.

3. Bake for 35 to 45 minutes until a fork can easily pierce the squash. Remove from the oven and let cool to the touch.

4. Using a fork, gently scrape the flesh of the squash from the shell.

COOKING TIP: You can also cook spaghetti squash in a slow cooker. To do so, prick the outside of a whole squash with a fork several times and place in the slow cooker. Cover and cook on low for 4 to 6 hours. When tender, carefully remove the squash and set on a cutting board to cool. Once cool, cut in half, remove the seeds, and use a fork to remove the flesh.

Per serving: Calories 138; Total fat 8g; Saturated fat 1g; Cholesterol 0mg; Carbs 18g; Fiber 0g; Protein 2g; Sodium 160mg

ROASTED GARLIC BRUSSELS SPROUTS

FLARE SOOTHER | FATIGUE-FRIENDLY | CARDIO CARE | BONE BOOSTER

Brussels sprouts are a great vegetable for roasting, because their flavor and sweetness increases as the natural sugars caramelize. Here they are tossed with balsamic vinegar and olive oil for a great finished product that requires very little hands-on time.

SERVES 4

Prep time: 5 minutes

Cook time: 20 minutes

2 tablespoons extra-virgin olive oil

2 tablespoons balsamic vinegar

3 garlic cloves, minced

½ teaspoon sea salt

Freshly ground black pepper

1 pound Brussels sprouts, trimmed and halved

1. Preheat the oven to 425°F.

2. In a large bowl, mix the olive oil, vinegar, garlic, salt, and pepper. Toss with the Brussels sprouts.

3. Spread on a baking sheet and roast for 15 to 20 minutes, stirring once, until tender and browned.

COOKING TIP: Brussels sprouts reheat well, so always be sure to make a pound, even if it is only you eating them. You can easily enjoy these throughout the week as a side dish to many meals.

Per serving: Calories 114; Total fat 7g; Saturated fat 1g; Cholesterol 0mg; Carbs 11g; Fiber 4g; Protein 4g; Sodium 263mg

ROASTED RUTABAGA

FATIGUE-FRIENDLY | CARDIO CARE | BONE BOOSTER

Rutabaga is an often-overlooked vegetable. A cross between a turnip and cabbage, rutabaga has sweet golden flesh and is wonderful when roasted. To minimize prep work, look for small rutabagas (about the size of an orange), which have a thinner skin that doesn't need to be peeled. Just scrub under running water. If you're using large ones, though, you will need to peel them.

SERVES 4

Prep time: 5 minutes

Cook time: 25 minutes

1 pound rutabaga, cut into 1-inch cubes

2 tablespoons extra-virgin olive oil

½ teaspoon sea salt

Juice of 1 lime

2 tablespoons chopped fresh parsley

1. Preheat the oven to 425°F.

2. In a large bowl, toss the rutabaga with the olive oil and salt. Arrange on a baking sheet in a single layer.

3. Roast for 20 to 25 minutes, flipping once about halfway through, until tender and browned.

4. Sprinkle with the lime juice and parsley and toss well.

INGREDIENT TIP: Similar to other root vegetables, rutabaga helps improve digestion and detoxify the liver. Rutabagas look a lot like turnips but are distinguishable by their green and purple skin. They can be small like a turnip or as large as a cabbage.

Per serving: Calories 104; Total fat 7g; Saturated fat 1g; Cholesterol 0mg; Carbs 10g; Fiber 3g; Protein 2g; Sodium 258mg

GARLIC-ROASTED GREEN BEANS

FATIGUE-FRIENDLY | KIDNEY SUPPORT | CARDIO CARE | BONE BOOSTER

Fresh green beans, like many other vegetables, are even better after roasting. This is a great way to prepare them that gives you plenty of time to tidy up or focus on another dish, because once you get them in the oven, you are pretty much done.

SERVES 2

Prep time: 5 minutes

Cook time: 25 minutes

1 pound green
beans, trimmed

2 tablespoons coconut
oil, melted

¼ teaspoon sea salt

5 garlic cloves, minced

1. Preheat the oven to 400°F.

2. On a baking sheet, arrange the beans in a single layer. Drizzle the coconut oil over the beans. Sprinkle with the salt.

3. Roast for 20 minutes, stirring once halfway through. Sprinkle the garlic over the beans and cook for an additional 3 to 5 minutes until fragrant. Serve.

INGREDIENT TIP: There are many different varieties of green beans to try. Summer is the height of bean season, so be sure to experiment and find your favorites. Look around at farmers' markets and grocery stores for haricots vert, snap beans, string beans, wax beans, runner beans, and more.

Per serving: Calories 199; Total fat 14g; Saturated fat 12g; Cholesterol 0mg; Carbs 19g;
Fiber 8g; Protein 5g; Sodium 249mg

SAUTÉED MUSTARD GREENS

FLARE SOOTHER | FATIGUE-FRIENDLY | CARDIO CARE | BONE BOOSTER

Mustard greens are one of the most pungent greens, but when cooked, the strong mustard oil that gives them their bite dissipates. A powerful high-nutrient vegetable, these flavorful greens add so much to a meal with just a quick sauté in a bit of garlic and lemon juice.

SERVES 4

Prep time: 5 minutes

Cook time: 15 minutes

2 tablespoons extra-virgin olive oil

2 pounds mustard greens, chopped

3 garlic cloves, thinly sliced

Juice of ¼ lemon

½ teaspoon sea salt

¼ teaspoon freshly ground black pepper

1. In a Dutch oven or covered skillet or sauté pan, heat the oil over medium-high heat. Add the mustard greens in batches, stirring until wilted before adding more greens.

2. Stir in the garlic and cook for 30 seconds until fragrant.

3. Cover and reduce the heat to medium. Cook, stirring occasionally, for 10 minutes until the greens are tender.

4. Add the lemon juice and stir well. Season with salt and pepper.

SUBSTITUTION TIP: You can use other hearty greens, such as kale or collards, in place of mustard greens in this recipe.

Per serving: Calories 125; Total fat 8g; Saturated fat 1g; Cholesterol 0mg; Carbs 12g; Fiber 8g; Protein 6g; Sodium 293mg

SLOW-COOKED COLLARD GREENS

FLARE SOOTHER | **FATIGUE-FRIENDLY** | **CARDIO CARE** | **BONE BOOSTER**

Collard greens are a Southern classic, and when cooked in the slow cooker, they couldn't be any easier to prepare. Smoked turkey is a lower-fat alternative to the more traditional ham hock that is used to flavor greens, yet it still brings the rich, meaty flavor.

SERVES 4

Prep time: 10 minutes

Cook time: 3 to 6 hours

2 pounds collard greens, thick stems removed, leaves chopped

1 smoked turkey neck

1 onion, chopped

3 garlic cloves, minced

6 cups water

Vinegar

Sea salt

1. In a slow cooker, combine the collard greens, turkey neck, onion, garlic, and water.

2. Cover and cook on low for 6 hours or on high for 3 hours.

3. Remove the turkey neck. Let it cool to the touch, then remove and shred the meat. Return the meat to the slow cooker.

4. Taste and season with vinegar and salt. Serve in a bowl with some of the liquid spooned over.

SUBSTITUTION TIP: Use a mixture of other firm greens that you have on hand to make this slow-cooked favorite. Kale, turnip greens, and mustard greens all hold up well to the long cook time of this recipe.

Per serving: Calories 85; Total fat 2g; Saturated fat 0g; Cholesterol 5mg, Carbs 16g; Fiber 8g; Protein 7g; Sodium 162mg

BRAISED MUSHROOMS

FLARE SOOTHER | FATIGUE-FRIENDLY | CARDIO CARE | BONE BOOSTER

Mushrooms can be so tasty on their own, with just a few aromatic seasonings to accentuate their unique flavor. This is an easy side that locks in a lot of flavor from the bone broth to help nourish your body. Serve these mushrooms with red meat or chicken for a perfect pairing.

SERVES 4

Prep time: 5 minutes

Cook time: 20 minutes

2 tablespoons extra-virgin olive oil

1 shallot, finely chopped

4 fresh sage leaves, thinly sliced

1 cup Chicken Bone Broth (page 151)

¼ teaspoon sea salt

Freshly ground black pepper

1 pound brown mushrooms, wiped clean

1. In a large skillet, heat the olive oil over medium-high heat.

2. Add the shallot and sage leaves and cook, stirring regularly, for about 2 minutes.

3. Add the broth, salt, and pepper, and bring to a simmer.

4. Add the mushrooms, reduce the heat to medium, cover, and cook for 6 minutes. Remove the lid and continue to cook for 8 to 10 additional minutes until tender.

SUBSTITUTION TIP: If you can get a variety of different mushrooms, try them here. Shiitake, oyster, porcini, and portabella mushrooms are all tasty when braised.

Per serving: Calories 95; Total fat 7g; Saturated fat 1g; Cholesterol 0mg; Carbs 5g; Fiber 1g; Protein 3g; Sodium 147mg

BRAISED FRESH TURNIPS AND GREENS

FLARE SOOTHER	FATIGUE-FRIENDLY	CARDIO CARE	BONE BOOSTER

Turnips are high in vitamins B and C and other nutrients, and have a delicate sweetness that is so wonderful in fresh salads and when cooked. Here the humble root is braised alongside its own greens and dressed up with coconut milk to create a creamy and hearty side dish.

SERVES 4

Prep time: 10 minutes

Cook time: 20 minutes

8 small turnips, with greens

1 tablespoon extra-virgin olive oil

½ cup Chicken Bone Broth (page 151)

¼ teaspoon sea salt

¼ cup canned coconut milk

1. Remove the greens from the turnips and finely chop. Cut the turnips in half lengthwise.

2. In a large skillet, heat the olive oil over medium heat. Place the turnips in the pan, cut-side down, and cook for 3 to 5 minutes until browned.

3. Flip the turnips and add the broth and salt. Bring to a simmer, cover, and cook for 6 minutes until the turnips are just starting to soften.

4. Add the greens and cook for 5 to 6 more minutes, stirring regularly, until the greens are wilted and the turnips are cooked through.

5. Stir in the coconut milk and serve.

SUBSTITUTION TIP: If you can't find turnips still attached to their greens, no problem. Buy loose turnips and substitute about 3 cups of chopped fresh spinach. Reduce the cooking time of the greens to 2 to 3 minutes, until the spinach wilts.

Per serving: Calories 136; Total fat 7g; Saturated fat 4g; Cholesterol 0mg; Carbs 17g; Fiber 4g; Protein 3g; Sodium 290mg

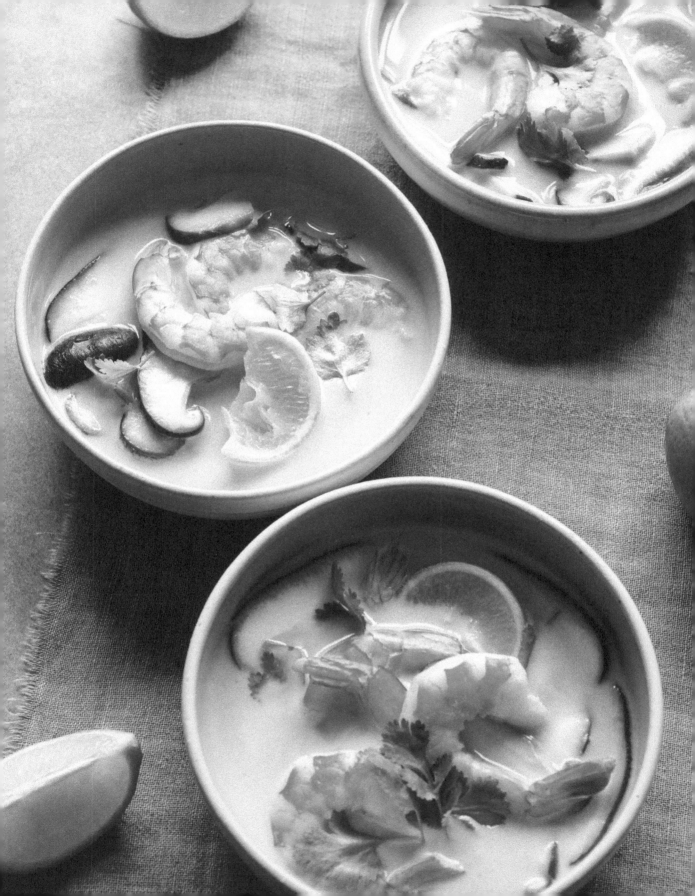

4

Salads and Soups

BALSAMIC WATERMELON SALAD

FLARE SOOTHER | FATIGUE-FRIENDLY | CARDIO CARE | BONE BOOSTER

Bitter arugula and sweet watermelon are a perfect pairing in this simple summer salad. Arugula is packed with vitamins A and C, folic acid, and calcium, and is a great digestive aid. Watermelon will keep you hydrated while supplying a dose of lycopene to support healthy vision.

SERVES 4

Prep time: 5 minutes

3 cups chopped watermelon

2 cups baby arugula

2 tablespoons Balsamic Vinaigrette (page 155)

1 tablespoon thinly sliced fresh mint leaves

In a large bowl, toss the watermelon, arugula, and vinaigrette. Garnish with the mint and serve.

SUBSTITUTION TIP: If you can't find or don't like arugula, substitute an equal amount of baby salad greens.

Per serving: Calories 67; Total fat 3g; Saturated fat 1g; Cholesterol 0mg; Carbs 10g; Fiber 1g; Protein 1g; Sodium 65mg

SPINACH AND MARINATED RED ONION SALAD

FLARE SOOTHER | FATIGUE-FRIENDLY | CARDIO CARE | BONE BOOSTER

It's amazing the difference that just 30 minutes of marinating makes to onions. When combined with fresh berries, you get a healthy serving of antioxidants in a wonderfully balanced fresh salad.

SERVES 2

Prep time: 5 minutes, plus 30 minutes to marinate

1 red onion, thinly sliced

2 tablespoons red wine vinegar

Sea salt

4 cups chopped spinach leaves

Juice of 1 lemon

1 garlic clove, minced

2 tablespoons extra-virgin olive oil

½ cup fresh berries (raspberries, strawberries, blueberries)

1. In a small bowl, combine the onion, vinegar, and a pinch of salt. Refrigerate for 30 minutes.

2. In a large bowl, toss the spinach with the lemon juice, garlic, and olive oil. Season with salt, and fold in the berries and onion.

SUBSTITUTION TIP: If you have Balsamic Vinaigrette (page 155) or Garlic-Cilantro Vinaigrette (page 156) on hand, you can use it to marinate the onion instead of the balsamic vinegar. Use ¼ cup to marinate the onion and omit the lemon juice, garlic, and olive oil.

Per serving: Calories 183; Total fat 15g; Saturated fat 2g; Cholesterol 0mg; Carbs 12g; Fiber 5g; Protein 3g; Sodium 173mg

CUCUMBER AVOCADO SALAD

Avocados are a wonderful source of monounsaturated fat, which accounts for 20 percent of their volume. Here the fruit is paired with crunchy cucumbers and marinated in an apple cider vinaigrette. It makes a perfect side salad for a summer meal.

SERVES 2

Prep time: 10 minutes,
plus 1 hour to marinate

1 tablespoon extra-virgin
olive oil

2 tablespoons apple
cider vinegar

1 tablespoon honey

½ teaspoon sea salt

2 large cucumbers,
thinly sliced

1 avocado, pitted, peeled,
and chopped

¼ cup chopped fresh cilantro

1. In a small bowl, whisk the olive oil, vinegar, honey, and salt.

2. In a medium bowl, toss the cucumbers with the dressing. Cover and refrigerate for at least 1 hour or as long as overnight.

3. Strain the liquid from the cucumbers, reserving it. Add the avocado and cilantro to the cucumbers and toss well. Drizzle with a couple of tablespoons of the reserved liquid just before serving.

SUBSTITUTION TIP: Don't have honey? No problem. Use pure maple syrup instead.

Per serving: Calories 285; Total fat 21g; Saturated fat 3g; Cholesterol 0mg; Carbs 27g; Fiber 8g; Protein 4g; Sodium 483mg

BROCCOLI AND OLIVE SALAD

FLARE SOOTHER | FATIGUE-FRIENDLY | CARDIO CARE | BONE BOOSTER

Broccoli contains nearly the same amount of calcium as milk and twice the amount of vitamin C as an orange! These are just two of the reasons you should include this cruciferous powerhouse in your diet as often as possible. Plan ahead so there's time for the salad to marinate for the most flavor. It keeps well, so you can pack it for lunches throughout the week.

SERVES 6

Prep time: 10 minutes,
plus 1 hour to marinate

Cook time: 5 minutes

1 pound broccoli florets, cut into bite-size pieces

¼ cup pitted and thinly sliced Kalamata olives

¼ cup thinly sliced red onion

2 tablespoons extra-virgin olive oil

2 tablespoons red wine vinegar

1 garlic clove, minced

1 teaspoon honey

¼ teaspoon sea salt

1. Bring a large pot of water to a boil over high heat. Fill a large bowl with cold water and add 10 to 12 ice cubes.

2. Blanch the broccoli in the boiling water for 1 to 2 minutes. Using a large slotted spoon or strainer, immediately transfer the broccoli to the ice water bath. Let rest for 2 to 3 minutes until cool. Drain.

3. In a large bowl, toss the broccoli, olives, and onion.

4. In a small bowl, whisk the olive oil, vinegar, garlic, honey, and salt to combine.

5. Toss the dressing with the broccoli mixture. Let marinate for at least 1 hour before serving, so the flavors mix.

COOKING TIP: While broccoli can be eaten raw, it is much easier for your body to digest when it is cooked. Blanching, the cooking style used here, quickly cooks the broccoli, then the ice-water bath abruptly halts the cooking process, so the broccoli is still bright green and firm but cooked just enough to allow for easier digestion.

Per serving: Calories 163; Total fat 13g; Saturated fat 2g; Cholesterol 0mg; Carbs 11g; Fiber 2g; Protein 2g; Sodium 624mg

NOTATO SALAD

FLARE SOOTHER | FATIGUE-FRIENDLY | CARDIO CARE | BONE BOOSTER

Don't feel left out of the picnic fun with this copycat potato salad, minus the potatoes. This healthy and easy salad is great as a side dish for grilled foods, and tastes fresh and fun year round.

SERVES 6

Prep time: 15 minutes, plus 1 hour to marinate

Cook time: 30 minutes

3 cups chopped turnip

3 cups chopped rutabaga

3 cups chopped daikon

1 small red onion, chopped

1 cucumber, peeled and chopped

2 celery stalks, chopped

2 tablespoons extra-virgin olive oil

½ teaspoon sea salt

1 tablespoon chopped fresh dill

2 tablespoons freshly squeezed lemon juice

¼ cup coconut cream

1. In a steamer, cook the turnip and rutabaga for 20 minutes until fork tender. Remove and rinse under cold water. Steam the daikon for 8 to 10 minutes until fork tender. Rinse under cold water.

2. In a large bowl, mix the daikon, turnip, rutabaga, onion, cucumber, and celery.

3. In a small bowl, whisk the olive oil, salt, dill, lemon juice, and coconut cream. Pour over the salad and stir to combine.

4. Refrigerate for at least 1 hour before serving.

INGREDIENT TIP: Coconut cream is the thick paste-like cream that separates and rises to the top of a can of coconut milk. To make it easier to remove the coconut cream from coconut milk, refrigerate a can of coconut milk overnight; the cream will rise to the top and harden. Open the can without shaking and scoop the cream from the top.

Per serving: Calories 152; Total fat 7g; Saturated fat 3g; Cholesterol 0mg; Carbs 22g; Fiber 5g; Protein 3g; Sodium 249mg

ROASTED BEET SALAD

The pigment that gives beets their color, betacyanin, is a powerful anti-inflammatory antioxidant, making them a wonderful vegetable to add to your regular repertoire. This delicious salad is super easy to make, though you will need to plan a little time for roasting and marinating the beets first. Do this simple prep work the night before, then toss the salad together when you are ready to serve. This hands-off method locks in a lot of flavor and couldn't be easier.

SERVES 6

Prep time: 10 minutes,
plus 2 hours to marinate

Cook time: 1 hour

6 medium beets

1 tablespoon extra-virgin
olive oil

½ cup Balsamic Vinaigrette
(page 155)

2 cups mixed baby
salad greens

¼ cup thinly sliced red onion

1. Preheat the oven to 350°F.

2. Wash the beets well and trim the ends. Toss with the olive oil and arrange the beets in a baking pan. Cover with aluminum foil and roast for 1 hour until the beets are tender. Let cool to the touch.

3. Peel and dice the beets. In a large bowl, combine the beets and vinaigrette. Toss to coat and then refrigerate for at least 2 hours or as long as overnight.

4. Strain the beets, reserving the vinaigrette. Toss the beets with the salad greens and onion. Drizzle the salad with 2 tablespoons of the reserved vinaigrette and toss well.

VARIATION TIP: If you have an Instant Pot or another brand of electric pressure cooker, you can save time by cooking the beets in the cooker. Add 1 cup of water and a trivet to the pressure cooker, and arrange the beets on the trivet. Cook on high pressure for 15 minutes, and when cooking is complete, let the pressure release naturally for 10 minutes and quick release any remaining pressure.

Per serving: Calories 166; Total fat 11g; Saturated fat 2g; Cholesterol 0mg; Carbs 16g; Fiber 3g; Protein 3g; Sodium 285mg

SWEET POTATO AND GREENS SALAD

FLARE SOOTHER | FATIGUE-FRIENDLY | CARDIO CARE | BONE BOOSTER

This hearty salad can easily be a side dish for a meat main course, or it can stand on its own for a light lunch. The coconut milk gives it a luxurious richness, and a generous helping of kale offers plenty of bone-strengthening calcium.

SERVES 4

Prep time: 5 minutes

Cook time: 40 minutes

2 pounds sweet potatoes, quartered lengthwise and cut into ½-inch slices

3 garlic cloves, minced

4 tablespoons melted coconut oil, divided

Sea salt

Freshly ground black pepper

8 cups stemmed and chopped kale

½ cup full-fat coconut milk

1. Preheat the oven to 400°F. Line a baking sheet with parchment paper.

2. In a large bowl, toss the sweet potatoes, garlic, and 2 tablespoons of the coconut oil. Arrange the pieces on the baking sheet in a single layer. Season with salt and pepper. Bake for 30 to 40 minutes, flipping once about halfway through, until the potatoes begin to brown.

3. While the sweet potatoes are cooking, in a large skillet, heat the remaining 2 tablespoons of coconut oil. Working in batches, add the kale to the skillet, stirring until it wilts before adding more kale. Cook for about 5 minutes until the kale is wilted but still bright green.

4. Pour in the coconut milk and stir well. Season with salt and pepper.

5. In a serving dish, mix together the kale and sweet potatoes. Serve warm.

SUBSTITUTION TIP: Other greens, such as collard greens, turnip greens, and mustard greens, all work well in this recipe.

Per serving: Calories 451; Total fat 21g; Saturated fat 18g; Cholesterol 0mg; Carbs 62g; Fiber 10g; Protein 8g; Sodium 246mg

SHRIMP, PINEAPPLE, AND CUCUMBER SALAD

FATIGUE-FRIENDLY | KIDNEY SUPPORT | CARDIO CARE

This salad will work as a main course, and you can have it on the table even quicker by forgoing the fresh pineapple and using canned. Buy a 20-ounce can of pineapple; just make sure that it is canned in its own juices and not a syrup (and make sure to drain it first). The mixture of lime juice, fish sauce, and cilantro makes this a refreshing sweet-and-sour dish, especially on a hot summer day.

SERVES 4

Prep time: 5 minutes

Cook time: 5 minutes

1 pound shrimp, shelled and deveined

Sea salt

2 cups diced pineapple

2 cucumbers, seeded and diced

¼ cup thinly sliced red onion

1 tablespoon fish sauce

1 tablespoon extra-virgin olive oil

Juice from 1 lime

Cilantro, for garnish

1. Preheat the oven to broil.

2. Lightly season the shrimp with salt and arrange on a baking sheet. Broil the shrimp for 2 to 3 minutes on each side, flipping once, until the shrimp are opaque and cooked through.

3. In a large bowl, toss the shrimp, pineapple, cucumber, and onion.

4. In a small bowl, whisk together the fish sauce, olive oil, and lime juice. Drizzle the sauce over the salad and toss to serve. Garnish with cilantro.

INGREDIENT TIP: Fish sauce is a condiment made from salted and fermented fish. Pungent and savory, it is a staple flavoring in many dishes from Southeast Asia. It can be found in the Asian section of many large grocery stores and at Asian markets.

Per serving: Calories 221; Total fat 6g; Saturated fat 1g; Cholesterol 170mg; Carbs 18g; Fiber 2g; Protein 25g; Sodium 522mg

CABBAGE AND BACON SLAW

FATIGUE-FRIENDLY | BONE BOOSTER

This salad goes with just about any dish and keeps well in the refrigerator, so I suggest you make a full recipe even if it seems like a lot. Cabbage is a strong antioxidant and is loaded with vitamin C. Cooked lightly, as in this salad, it is sweet, tender, and delicious.

SERVES 8

Prep time: 10 minutes

Cook time: 10 minutes

4 bacon slices, chopped

1 teaspoon honey

¼ cup apple cider vinegar

4 scallions, thinly sliced

1 small green cabbage (about 2 pounds), cored and shredded

Sea salt

1. In a large skillet over medium-high heat, cook the bacon, stirring regularly, for 6 to 8 minutes until it is cooked and browned. Transfer the bacon to a plate lined with paper towels, leaving the bacon grease in the pan.

2. In a small bowl, stir the honey into the vinegar. Add the scallions and set aside.

3. Add the cabbage to the skillet in batches, stirring a few times before adding more cabbage. Stir for 2 to 3 minutes until the cabbage becomes slightly tender.

4. Pour in the vinegar mixture and toss to combine. Stir the bacon back into the salad and season with salt, if necessary. Serve warm.

SUBSTITUTION TIP: If you want to skip the chopping, substitute two (14-ounce) packages of shredded cabbage. Use a mixture of red and green cabbage for added color, if possible.

Per serving: Calories 86; Total fat 4g; Saturated fat 1g; Cholesterol 10mg; Carbs 8g; Fiber 3g; Protein 5g; Sodium 273mg

BEET-COCONUT SOUP

FLARE SOOTHER | FATIGUE-FRIENDLY | CARDIO CARE | BONE BOOSTER

Beets have a lovely sweetness, and when paired with rich coconut milk, they are sublime. This bright soup is a great change of pace and perfect to liven a dreary day. Beets are detoxifying to the body and a natural anti-inflammatory, making them a wonderful addition to your diet.

SERVES 4

Prep time: 5 minutes

Cook time: 25 minutes

1 tablespoon extra-virgin olive oil

1 small onion, chopped

2 garlic cloves, minced

3 medium red beets, peeled and chopped into ½-inch pieces

4 cups Vegetable Broth (page 150) or Chicken Bone Broth (page 151)

1 (14-ounce) can coconut milk

1 teaspoon sea salt

1. In a large pot, heat the olive oil over medium-high heat and cook the onion for 3 to 5 minutes until softened. Add the garlic and cook until fragrant, about 30 seconds more.

2. Add the beets and broth. Bring to a boil, reduce the heat to medium-low, cover, and simmer until the beets are tender, about 20 minutes.

3. Using an immersion blender or a regular blender, purée the soup. Add the coconut milk and season with salt. Stir until mixed through.

INGREDIENT TIP: If you can get baby beets, use them here and you can skip the peeling, saving you a bit of work. Alternatively, cooked beets are showing up increasingly often in the produce section of grocery stores. To use these, simply chop and bring to a simmer in step 2, until they are heated through, then proceed with puréeing the soup.

Per serving: Calories 321; Total fat 27g; Saturated fat 22g; Cholesterol 0mg; Carbs 21g; Fiber 5g; Protein 4g; Sodium 581mg

CREAMY BROCCOLI SOUP

FLARE SOOTHER | FATIGUE-FRIENDLY | CARDIO CARE | BONE BOOSTER

Your taste buds and body will love this allergen-free version of the classic soup. Using coconut milk for creaminess and bone broth for its base, this soup is loaded with healthy fats and feel-good flavor without the dairy.

SERVES 4

Prep time: 5 minutes

Cook time: 20 minutes

1 tablespoon extra-virgin olive oil

1 small onion, chopped

2 garlic cloves, minced

4 cups broccoli florets

3 cups Chicken Bone Broth (page 151) or Beef Bone Broth (page 152)

¾ cup coconut milk

1 teaspoon sea salt

1. In a large pot, heat the olive oil over medium heat. Cook the onion for 3 to 5 minutes until softened. Add the garlic and cook until fragrant, about 30 seconds more.

2. Add the broccoli and bone broth. Bring to a boil, reduce the heat to medium-low, cover, and simmer for 10 to 15 minutes until the broccoli is fork tender.

3. Using an immersion blender or in a traditional blender, purée the soup. Add the coconut milk and season with salt. Stir over medium heat until heated through.

SUBSTITUTION TIP: Use this recipe as a base for a number of veggie soups—as many as your imagination can reach. Substitute cauliflower, spinach, your favorite greens, or any other leafy or cruciferous vegetable you like.

Per serving: Calories 181; Total fat 15g; Saturated fat 10g; Cholesterol 0mg; Carbs 11g; Fiber 4g; Protein 5g; Sodium 573mg

CREAM OF MUSHROOM SOUP

FLARE SOOTHER | FATIGUE-FRIENDLY | CARDIO CARE | BONE BOOSTER

Mushroom lovers will enjoy this soup for its rich and creamy flavor. If you are not a big mushroom fan, use this simple soup as a base to make a green bean casserole that sticks to your healthy diet and still tastes great.

SERVES 2

Prep time: 5 minutes

Cook time: 20 minutes

1 tablespoon extra-virgin olive oil

1 small onion, chopped

2 garlic cloves, minced

2½ cups chopped baby bella mushrooms

1½ cups Chicken Bone Broth (page 151) or Beef Bone Broth (page 152)

1 cup canned full-fat coconut milk

Sea salt

1. In a large pot, heat the olive oil over medium heat. Cook the onion for 3 to 5 minutes until softened. Add the garlic and cook until fragrant, about 30 seconds more.

2. Add the mushrooms and stir to combine. Continue to cook for about 5 minutes until the mushrooms are browned.

3. Pour in the bone broth and bring to a boil, reduce the heat to medium-low, cover, and simmer for about 12 minutes until the mushrooms are softened.

4. Using an immersion blender or in a traditional blender, purée the soup. Add the coconut milk and stir to combine. Season with salt before serving.

SUBSTITUTION TIP: For even more flavor, try making this soup with different mushrooms or a medley of mushrooms. Anything from classic brown mushrooms to shiitake, porcini, and oyster mushrooms can add a different flavor and enrich this soup.

Per serving: Calories 388; Total fat 36g; Saturated fat 26g; Cholesterol 0mg; Carbs 15g; Fiber 4g; Protein 8g; Sodium 176mg

BUTTERNUT SQUASH SOUP

FLARE SOOTHER | CARDIO CARE | BONE BOOSTER

Butternut squash is often prepared sweet, but this savory soup is every bit as delicious. Winter squash such as butternut are loaded with vitamins A and C, potassium, and magnesium, making them a great choice for a soup that is both warming and nourishing.

SERVES 4

Prep time: 10 minutes

Cook time: 25 minutes

1 tablespoon extra-virgin olive oil

1 medium onion, chopped

1 medium butternut squash, peeled, seeded, and chopped

3 cups Chicken Bone Broth (page 151) or Beef Bone Broth (page 152)

1 cup canned full-fat coconut milk

1 teaspoon ground cinnamon

1 teaspoon ground turmeric

½ teaspoon sea salt

1. In a large pot, heat the olive oil over medium heat. Cook the onion for 3 to 5 minutes, stirring regularly, until softened.

2. Add the squash and broth. Bring to a boil, reduce the heat to medium-low, cover, and simmer for about 20 minutes until the squash is tender.

3. Using an immersion blender or in a traditional blender, purée the soup. Add the coconut milk, cinnamon, turmeric, and salt. Stir well and serve.

COOKING TIP: If you want to avoid chopping the squash, cook it whole in a slow cooker for 3 to 4 hours on high or for 5 to 6 hours on low. When done, let it cool to the touch, halve it, and remove the seeds. Scoop out the flesh and transfer to the broth in step 2 until just heated through, then purée the soup.

Per serving: Calories 284; Total fat 18g; Saturated fat 13g; Cholesterol 0mg; Carbs 32g; Fiber 7g; Protein 5g; Sodium 320mg

HEARTY VEGETABLE SOUP

FLARE SOOTHER | FATIGUE-FRIENDLY | CARDIO CARE | BONE BOOSTER

This is an easy soup to make that turns out delicious every time. You can customize it to your taste by swapping vegetables as you like, but be sure to try it with this combination at least once. Turnips lend a lovely hint of sweetness, along with a dose of vitamins B and C, potassium, phosphorus, and calcium. Be sure not to overcook them, as they can release a sulfurous aroma like cabbage.

SERVES 4

Prep time: 5 minutes

Cook time: 25 minutes

2 tablespoons extra-virgin olive oil

1 onion, chopped

3 garlic cloves, minced

2 carrots, chopped

2 celery stalks, chopped

2 turnips, peeled and chopped

4 cups Chicken Bone Broth (page 151) or Vegetable Broth (page 150)

1 teaspoon fresh thyme leaves

Sea salt

1. In a large pot, heat the olive oil over medium heat. Cook the onion for 3 to 5 minutes until softened. Add the garlic and cook until fragrant, about 30 seconds more.

2. Stir in the carrots, celery, and turnips. Continue to cook, stirring regularly, for 5 to 7 minutes, until the vegetables brown slightly.

3. Add the broth and thyme. Season with salt. Cook for 5 to 8 minutes longer, until the vegetables are tender.

SUBSTITUTION TIP: While thyme is a great seasoning in a soup such as this, it can easily be omitted or exchanged for whatever herbs you have on hand.

Per serving: Calories 116; Total fat 7g; Saturated fat 1g; Cholesterol 0mg; Carbs 12g; Fiber 3g; Protein 2g; Sodium 218mg

COCONUT LEMONGRASS SHRIMP SOUP

FLARE SOOTHER | FATIGUE-FRIENDLY | CARDIO CARE | BONE BOOSTER

Kissed with lemongrass, lime, and ginger, this flavorful broth is everything you need on a cold day. Similar to Thai tom kha soup but without the chiles, this soup is great on its own or as part of a larger meal. If you can't find fresh lemongrass, substitute the zest of one lemon.

SERVES 4

Prep time: 5 minutes

Cook time: 20 minutes

4 cups Chicken Bone Broth (page 151)

Zest and juice of 1 lime, divided

2 lemongrass stalks, white part only, thinly sliced

2-inch piece fresh ginger, peeled and chopped

2 cups water

8 ounces shrimp, peeled and deveined

2 cups thinly sliced shiitake mushrooms

1 (14-ounce) can full-fat coconut milk

1 tablespoon fish sauce

¼ cup chopped fresh cilantro leaves and stems

1. In a large pot over medium-high heat, combine the broth, lime zest, lemongrass, ginger, and water. Bring to a boil, reduce the heat to medium-low, and simmer for 15 minutes. Strain and discard the lemongrass and ginger. Return the broth to the pot.

2. Add the shrimp and mushrooms and cook over medium heat for 3 to 5 minutes until the shrimp is cooked through and pink.

3. Add the coconut milk, fish sauce, and lime juice. Serve garnished with the cilantro.

VARIATION TIP: If you want a little more bulk to the soup, add a cup of zucchini noodles to your serving bowl and just pour the hot soup on top.

Per serving: Calories 289; Total fat 24g; Saturated fat 21g; Cholesterol 60mg; Carbs 9g; Fiber 3g; Protein 13g; Sodium 599mg

CREAMY CLAM CHOWDER

FATIGUE-FRIENDLY

Creamy clam chowder gets a healthy makeover in this delicious soup. Sweet potatoes fill in for the usual white variety, and coconut milk and arrowroot powder create the creamy base this classic soup is known for. Canned clams make this recipe quick and simple, and they taste just as great as fresh.

SERVES 4

Prep time: 10 minutes

Cook time: 15 minutes

1 tablespoon extra-virgin olive oil

2 sweet potatoes, cut into ½-inch pieces

1 small onion, chopped

3 garlic cloves, minced

4 bacon slices, chopped

2 (5-ounce) cans clams

2 tablespoons arrowroot powder

1 (14-ounce) can coconut milk

½ teaspoon sea salt

2 scallions, chopped

1. In a large pot, heat the olive oil over medium-high heat. Add the sweet potatoes, onion, and garlic, and cook for 5 to 7 minutes until just starting to brown and soften. Add the bacon and cook until crisp, about 5 to 7 more minutes. Reduce the heat to medium-low.

2. Add the clams and their juices to the pot. Add the arrowroot powder and mix well until completely incorporated.

3. Whisk in the coconut milk and salt, and heat until the soup is just thickened but not boiling. Serve garnished with the scallions.

COOKING TIP: When cooking with coconut milk, be sure you don't let the liquid boil, as it can cause the coconut milk to separate. While this does not make the soup taste any different, the look of it can be unappetizing, as it can resemble curdled milk.

Per serving: Calories 562; Total fat 38g; Saturated fat 25g; Cholesterol 68mg; Carbs 30g; Fiber 5g; Protein 29g; Sodium 806mg

LEMON CHICKEN SOUP

FLARE SOOTHER	FATIGUE-FRIENDLY	KIDNEY SUPPORT	CARDIO CARE	BONE BOOSTER

This soup is similar to the Greek avgolemono soup, except instead of egg, as in the traditional version, this one uses cauliflower to thicken the soup. It is a fresh take on a classic soup that still locks in the best of flavors without sacrificing your diet.

SERVES 4

Prep time: 5 minutes

Cook time: 10 minutes

4 cups Chicken Bone Broth (page 151)

3 cups cauliflower florets

2 cups shredded cooked chicken

Juice of 3 lemons

Sea salt

Freshly ground black pepper

2 tablespoons chopped fresh dill

1. In a large pot over medium heat, combine the broth and cauliflower and bring to a simmer. Cook for 5 to 7 minutes until the cauliflower is tender.

2. Using an immersion blender or in a traditional blender, purée the cauliflower and broth.

3. Add the chicken to the soup in the pot and heat over medium heat. Add the lemon juice and season with salt and pepper.

4. Serve garnished with the dill.

COOKING TIP: If you don't have any cooked chicken on hand, poach a large chicken breast in the simmering broth until cooked through, 10 to 15 minutes, and remove it to shred before blending the soup.

Per serving: Calories 141; Total fat 2g; Saturated fat 1g; Cholesterol 54mg; Carbs 6g; Fiber 2g; Protein 23g; Sodium 221mg

HOMESTYLE CHICKEN AND VEGETABLE SOUP

FLARE SOOTHER | FATIGUE-FRIENDLY | KIDNEY SUPPORT | CARDIO CARE | BONE BOOSTER

The classic taste of chicken soup is always such a comfort. Make it yourself with minimal prep in this simple soup that is loaded with flavor. Like many of the other soups in this book, you can customize the vegetables as desired, but this is a nutritious combination that plays on what you likely have on hand at home, making it all the easier.

SERVES 6

Prep time: 10 minutes

Cook time: 25 minutes

1 tablespoon extra-virgin olive oil

1 small onion, chopped

4 cups Chicken Bone Broth (page 151)

2 cups water

2 boneless, skinless chicken breasts

2 carrots, cut into ¼-inch slices

2 celery stalks, cut into ¼-inch slices

Sea salt

1. In a large pot, heat the olive oil over medium heat. Cook the onion for 5 to 7 minutes until softened.

2. Add the broth and water. Raise the heat to high and bring to a boil. Add the chicken breasts, carrots, and celery and reduce the heat to a simmer. Cook for 14 to 16 minutes until the vegetables are tender and the chicken is cooked through.

3. Remove the chicken and, using two forks, shred the chicken. Return it to the soup.

4. Season with salt and serve hot.

INGREDIENT TIP: If you have cooked chicken, add it in step 3 after the vegetables are cooked.

Per serving: Calories 91; Total fat 3g; Saturated fat 0g; Cholesterol 27mg; Carbs 4g; Fiber 1g; Protein 12g; Sodium 149mg

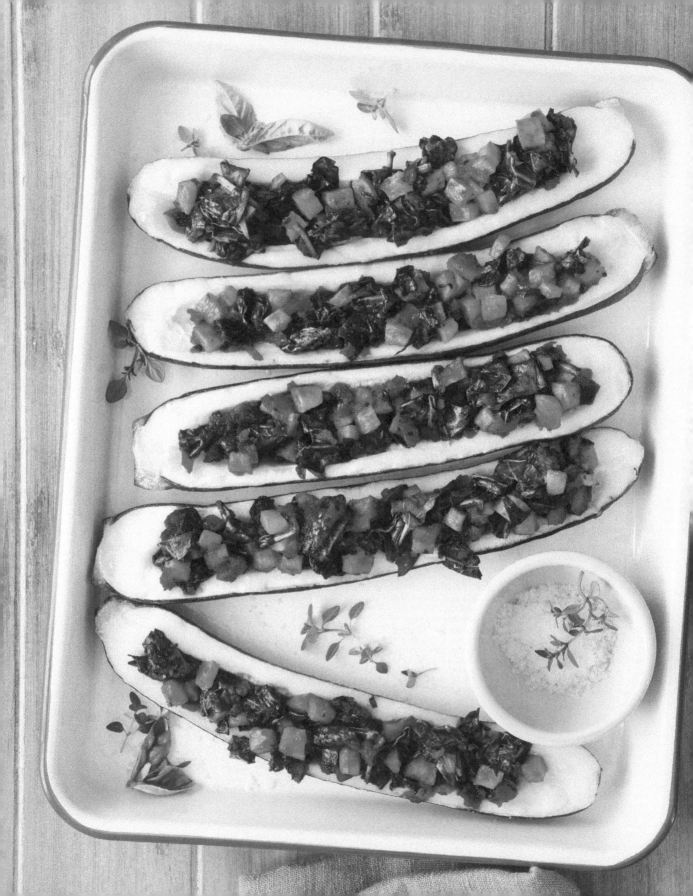

5

Plant-Based Meals

ZUCCHINI NOODLE PESTO

| FLARE SOOTHER | FATIGUE-FRIENDLY | CARDIO CARE | BONE BOOSTER |

Zucchini noodles are so wonderful because of their simplicity and versatility. You can cook them briefly for tenderness—but when mixed with a fresh pesto, I think they taste best raw, where they keep a slightly firmer texture.

SERVES 2

Prep time: 10 minutes

2 medium zucchini

1 recipe Nut-Free Basil Pesto (page 164)

1. Using a spiralizer or vegetable peeler, cut the zucchini into veggie "noodles."

2. In a large bowl, toss with the pesto sauce and serve.

INGREDIENT TIP: If you are too tired to make the noodles, look in the packaged produce section of your grocery store. Many grocery stores now sell noodles made from different kinds of squash and other veggies.

Per serving: Calories 395; Total fat 36g; Saturated fat 6g; Cholesterol 0mg; Carbs 17g; Fiber 6g; Protein 14g; Sodium 266mg

ZUCCHINI-CARROT FRITTERS

Fritters are a great way to eat more vegetables. Serve these fritters with Creamy Egg-Free Mayo (page 154) for dipping.

SERVES 4

Prep time: 10 minutes

Cook time: 10 minutes

1 medium zucchini, grated

1 medium carrot, grated

3 scallions, thinly sliced

2 garlic cloves, minced

3 tablespoons coconut flour

½ teaspoon sea salt

1 tablespoon coconut oil

1. In a medium bowl, mix the zucchini, carrot, scallions, garlic, coconut flour, and salt. Form into four patties.

2. Heat the coconut oil in a large skillet over medium heat. Fry the fritters on each side for 3 to 4 minutes, flipping once, until browned and crisp. Remove from the skillet and serve hot.

VARIATION TIP: These can be baked if you prefer. Line a baking sheet with parchment paper and bake in a 400°F oven for 20 to 25 minutes, flipping once about halfway through.

Per serving: Calories 94; Total fat 5g; Saturated fat 4g; Cholesterol 0mg; Carbs 12g; Fiber 6g; Protein 3g; Sodium 251mg

VEGGIE NUGGETS

FLARE SOOTHER | FATIGUE-FRIENDLY | KIDNEY SUPPORT | CARDIO CARE

It's not hard to eat all your daily servings of vegetables when you have these nuggets to munch on. Cauliflower, zucchini, and scallions come together for tasty, crisp nuggets that are perfect for dipping.

SERVES 2

Prep time: 10 minutes

Cook time: 35 minutes

Coconut oil, for greasing

1 cup shredded zucchini

1 cup riced cauliflower

2 scallions, thinly sliced

¼ cup coconut flour

¼ teaspoon sea salt

3 tablespoons coconut oil

1. Preheat the oven to 400°F. Line a baking sheet with parchment paper and lightly grease the paper with coconut oil.

2. Place the zucchini and cauliflower in a clean dishtowel and wring it out to remove as much liquid as possible.

3. In a large bowl, combine the zucchini, cauliflower, scallions, coconut flour, and salt. Mix well.

4. Add the coconut oil and mix well. Form into 10 to 12 small nuggets and place them on the prepared baking sheet. Bake for 25 minutes, flip, and continue to bake for 10 more minutes until crisp.

COOKING TIP: Be sure to use a metal spatula when flipping. The nuggets will be fragile when you flip them and will firm up as they crisp.

Per serving: Calories 322; Total fat 24g; Saturated fat 20g; Cholesterol 0mg; Carbs 26g; Fiber 14g; Protein 6g; Sodium 257mg

STUFFED ZUCCHINI BOATS

| FLARE SOOTHER | FATIGUE-FRIENDLY | CARDIO CARE | BONE BOOSTER |

These veggie-stuffed zucchini boats are a perfect summertime meal. Make the sweet potato–spinach filling while the zucchini cook and this simple, light meal comes together quickly.

SERVES 4

Prep time: 10 minutes

Cook time: 20 minutes

4 medium zucchini, halved lengthwise

2 tablespoons melted coconut oil, divided

Sea salt

3 garlic cloves, minced

1 small sweet potato, chopped

4 cups chopped spinach

½ cup Tomato-Free Marinara Sauce (page 165)

1. Preheat the oven to 400°F.

2. Scoop the seeds and flesh from the zucchini so that the shell is just ½ inch thick. Brush the inside of the zucchini shells with 1 tablespoon of the coconut oil. Season with salt.

3. On a baking sheet, arrange the zucchini cut-side up. Bake for 15 minutes until browned but not mushy.

4. While the squash is cooking, heat the remaining 1 tablespoon of coconut oil in a large skillet over medium-high heat. Cook the garlic for about 1 minute, stirring constantly, until fragrant and browned.

5. Add the sweet potato and cook for 10 to 15 minutes until tender. Stir in the spinach, a handful at a time, waiting until it wilts to add more. Stir in the marinara sauce.

6. Spoon the mixture into the zucchini shells. Adjust the oven to broil.

7. Broil for 2 to 3 minutes on the top rack until the tops are browned.

SUBSTITUTION TIP: Straightneck yellow summer squash also work well in this recipe. You may need to add a couple of minutes to the cooking time in step 3 for tenderness.

Per serving: Calories 152; Total fat 7g; Saturated fat 6g; Cholesterol 0mg; Carbs 17g; Fiber 4g; Protein 4g; Sodium 158mg

PAD THAI ZUCCHINI NOODLES

| FLARE SOOTHER | FATIGUE-FRIENDLY | KIDNEY SUPPORT | CARDIO CARE |

Pad Thai just got a whole lot healthier with this veggie-forward remake that exchanges the more typical rice noodles for those made from zucchini.

SERVES 4

Prep time: 15 minutes

Cook time: 5 minutes

2 tablespoons freshly squeezed lime juice

2 tablespoons fish sauce

1 teaspoon honey

2 medium zucchini

2 tablespoons extra-virgin olive oil, divided

3 garlic cloves, minced

3 scallions, sliced

1 cup thinly sliced snow peas

2 cups bean sprouts

¼ cup chopped cilantro leaves and stems

Lime wedges, for serving

1. In a small bowl, whisk together the lime juice, fish sauce, and honey.

2. Using a spiralizer, mandoline, or vegetable peeler, cut the zucchini into noodles.

3. In a large skillet over medium heat, heat 1 tablespoon of the olive oil and cook the zucchini noodles for 2 to 3 minutes until just tender. Remove from the skillet and set aside.

4. Heat the remaining 1 tablespoon of olive oil over medium heat. Add the garlic and cook until fragrant, about 30 seconds. Add the scallions and peas and cook for 1 minute until still crisp tender. Add the bean sprouts and stir well.

5. Return the zucchini noodles to the skillet and stir well. Pour the sauce into the skillet and stir to mix. Serve, topped with the cilantro and lime wedges on the side.

SUBSTITUTION TIP: Butternut squash noodles can be a fun (and colorful!) alternative to zucchini noodles in this recipe. Look for them in the prepared produce section at health food stores.

Per serving: Calories 149; Total fat 8g; Saturated fat 1g; Cholesterol 0mg; Carbs 17g; Fiber 4g; Protein 6g; Sodium 713mg

VEGGIE CAULI-RICE STIR-FRY

FLARE SOOTHER | FATIGUE-FRIENDLY | CARDIO CARE | BONE BOOSTER

Cauliflower rice has been around for a while, but one of my favorite ways to eat it is as fried "rice." Carrots, zucchini, and mushrooms come together for a delicious, simple, and filling rice-like stir-fry.

SERVES 4

Prep time: 10 minutes

Cook time: 15 minutes

2 tablespoons coconut aminos

½ teaspoon ground turmeric

1 cauliflower head, cut into florets

2 tablespoons coconut oil

1 medium onion, chopped

3 garlic cloves, minced

1-inch piece fresh ginger, minced

1 carrot, finely diced

1 zucchini, finely diced

1 cup finely chopped mushrooms

1. In a small bowl, whisk the coconut aminos and turmeric. Set aside.

2. In a food processor, pulse the cauliflower until it resembles rice.

3. In a large skillet, heat the coconut oil over medium heat. Cook the onion, garlic, and ginger, stirring constantly, for about 5 minutes until the onion is translucent.

4. Add the carrot, zucchini, and mushrooms, and continue to cook for 5 minutes until the vegetables are just fork tender. Stir in the cauliflower rice and the coconut aminos mixture and mix well. Continue to stir for 2 to 3 minutes until the cauliflower is heated through and just barely tender.

INGREDIENT TIP: To save time, you can buy pre-riced bags of cauliflower in the packaged produce section or frozen foods section of many grocery stores.

Per serving: Calories 116; Total fat 7g; Saturated fat 6g; Cholesterol 0mg; Carbs 12g; Fiber 4g; Protein 3g; Sodium 46mg

SQUASH STUFFED WITH CAULI-RICE AND VEGETABLES

| FLARE SOOTHER | FATIGUE-FRIENDLY | CARDIO CARE | BONE BOOSTER |

Winter squash is the perfect vehicle for stuffing, and here it is loaded with vegetables and topped off with antioxidant-rich dried cherries.

SERVES 4

Prep time: 10 minutes

Cook time: 25 minutes

2 tablespoons extra-virgin olive oil, divided

2 delicata squash, cut in half lengthwise and seeded

1 cauliflower head, cut into florets

1 onion, chopped

4 cups stemmed and chopped kale

½ teaspoon sea salt

¼ cup dried unsweetened cherries

1. Preheat the oven to 400°F.

2. Rub 1 tablespoon of the olive oil on both sides of the squash. Arrange the squash on a baking sheet, cut-sides up, and roast for 25 minutes until tender.

3. While the squash is cooking, in a food processor, pulse the cauliflower until it resembles rice.

4. In a large skillet, heat the remaining 1 tablespoon of olive oil over medium heat. Add the onion and cook for 3 to 5 minutes until softened. Add the cauliflower and kale and cook for 3 to 5 more minutes until the cauliflower and kale are tender. Stir in the salt and cherries.

5. Scoop the cauliflower rice into the cooked squash and serve warm.

SUBSTITUTION TIP: If you can't find delicata squash, other small varieties that work well include acorn and buttercup squash.

Per serving: Calories 234; Total fat 8g; Saturated fat 1g; Cholesterol 0mg; Carbs 41g; Fiber 9g; Protein 7g; Sodium 315mg

VEGGIE BURRITO BOWL

In this reimagined burrito bowl loaded with sweet potatoes and cauliflower, everything comes together seamlessly. Coconut cream, cilantro, and scallions provide fresh and bright flavors, and the turmeric-kissed sweet potatoes are filling and delicious. This reheats well for weekday lunches.

SERVES 4

Prep time: 5 minutes

2 sweet potatoes, chopped

3 tablespoons melted coconut oil, divided

1 teaspoon ground turmeric

1 teaspoon sea salt, divided

1 small cauliflower head

½ cup full-fat coconut cream

¼ cup chopped fresh cilantro

3 scallions, sliced

1 teaspoon onion powder

½ teaspoon garlic powder

1 romaine lettuce head, chopped

½ cup pitted and sliced black olives

1. Preheat the oven to 425°F. Line a baking sheet with parchment paper.

2. In a large bowl, toss the sweet potatoes with 2 tablespoons of the coconut oil, the turmeric, and ¼ teaspoon of the salt. Arrange in a single layer on the baking sheet. Cook for 20 to 25 minutes, flipping once about halfway through, until browned and tender.

3. While the potatoes are cooking, in a food processor, pulse the cauliflower until it resembles rice.

4. In a large skillet, heat the remaining 1 tablespoon of coconut oil over medium heat, and add the cauliflower. Cook for 6 to 8 minutes, covered, stirring regularly. When the cauliflower is tender, add the coconut cream, cilantro, scallions, onion powder, remaining salt, and garlic powder. Mix well.

5. In serving bowls, layer the lettuce, cauliflower rice, and sweet potatoes. Garnish with the olives.

INGREDIENT TIP: For the coconut cream used in this recipe or any other, you can either scrape the cream from the top of a jar of coconut milk without shaking, or you can buy a can of coconut cream at a specialty store, health food store, or Asian or Caribbean market. If you're buying canned coconut cream, look for a brand that is unsweetened.

Per serving: Calories 325; Total fat 17g; Saturated fat 15g; Cholesterol 0mg; Carbs 41g; Fiber 5g; Protein 4g; Sodium 637mg

CAULIFLOWER-MUSHROOM "RISOTTO"

FLARE SOOTHER | **FATIGUE-FRIENDLY** | **BONE BOOSTER**

This creamy "risotto" is another great way that cauliflower can be used like rice. Traditionally made with Arborio rice, this remade classic is loaded with bone-supporting broth and made creamy with coconut cream instead of cheese. Mushrooms give it a meaty feel, and best of all, your belly will feel great after eating this rich dish.

SERVES 4

Prep time: 10 minutes

Cook time: 15 minutes

1 small cauliflower head, cut into florets

2 tablespoons extra-virgin olive oil

1 shallot, chopped

2 cups finely chopped brown mushrooms

3 garlic cloves, minced

½ cup Chicken Bone Broth (page 151) or Vegetable Broth (page 150)

2 tablespoons coconut cream

Sea salt

1. In a food processor, pulse the cauliflower until it resembles rice.

2. In a medium pot, heat the olive oil over medium heat. Add the shallot and cook for 3 minutes until just softened. Add the mushrooms and garlic, and cook for 3 to 4 minutes until the mushrooms begin to brown.

3. Add the cauliflower and stir to combine. Then add the broth, a few tablespoons at a time, letting the broth cook off before adding more.

4. When you add the last few tablespoons of broth, add the coconut cream, stir, then cover the pot to steam for 1 to 2 minutes until tender. Season with salt and serve.

COOKING TIP: Save time by ricing a couple of heads of cauliflower at once to have on hand for quick meal prep. Store in an airtight container in the refrigerator for 3 to 4 days. When you are ready to use, proceed with step 2.

Per serving: Calories 124; Total fat 9g; Saturated fat 3g; Cholesterol 0mg; Carbs 11g; Fiber 2g; Protein 3g; Sodium 96mg

MUSHROOM STROGANOFF OVER MASHED CAULIFLOWER

FLARE SOOTHER | FATIGUE-FRIENDLY | BONE BOOSTER

Stroganoff is a comfort-food superstar, and even without the noodles, this dish is a winner. Look for brown mushrooms, such as cremini or baby portabella, as they are commonly known. Though the flavor is similar to white mushrooms, brown mushrooms will create a beautiful dark stroganoff sauce.

SERVES 4

Prep time: 10 minutes

Cook time: 20 minutes

1 cauliflower head, cut into florets

3 tablespoons extra-virgin olive oil

1 pound sliced brown mushrooms

1 onion, sliced

½ teaspoon garlic powder

Sea salt

1 cup Chicken Bone Broth (page 151), Beef Bone Broth (page 152), or Vegetable Broth (page 150)

1 cup coconut cream

2 tablespoons chopped fresh parsley

1. In a steamer, cook the cauliflower until tender, 5 to 10 minutes, depending on the size of the florets.

2. Meanwhile, in a large skillet, heat the olive oil over medium heat. Cook the mushrooms and onion for 5 to 7 minutes until translucent. Season with the garlic powder and salt.

3. Stir in the broth, taste, and season with more salt if needed. Stir in the coconut cream and continue to stir until heated through.

4. Using a potato masher, mash the cauliflower. Serve the cauliflower topped with the mushroom mixture and parsley.

SUBSTITUTION TIP: You can use another mashed vegetable here in place of the cauliflower. Turnips, rutabaga, parsnips, sweet potatoes, or a combination of a couple all work well as a vegetable mash with stroganoff.

Per serving: Calories 436; Total fat 23g; Saturated fat 13g; Cholesterol 0mg; Carbs 55g; Fiber 5g; Protein 7g; Sodium 160mg

SAVORY VEGETABLE TART

FATIGUE-FRIENDLY | CARDIO CARE | BONE BOOSTER

This vegetable tart uses a mixture of arrowroot powder and coconut flour to form a bed for the flavorful mix of scallions, mushrooms, artichoke hearts, and olives. Pesto brings the main flavor component to the dish. Enjoy this with salad for a nice lunch or serve it alongside a meat main dish for a more filling meal.

SERVES 4

Prep time: 15 minutes

Cook time: 25 minutes

1 cup arrowroot powder

½ cup coconut flour

½ teaspoon sea salt

⅓ cup coconut oil

¼ cup Nut-Free Basil Pesto (page 164)

3 scallions, sliced

1 cup sliced mushrooms

1 cup chopped artichoke hearts

½ cup sliced green or black olives

Sea salt

1. Preheat the oven to 400°F.

2. In a food processor, pulse the arrowroot powder, coconut flour, salt, and coconut oil until crumbly. Add ice-cold water, a tablespoon at a time, pulsing between each addition, until a dough forms.

3. Transfer the dough to a 9-inch pie or tart pan and press down into the pan. Prick the dough all over with a fork. Bake for 12 to 14 minutes until browned.

4. Spread the pesto sauce on the bottom of the tart. Top with the scallions, mushrooms, artichoke hearts, and olives. Season lightly with salt.

5. Bake for 10 to 12 minutes until heated through and the mushrooms and artichokes are lightly browned.

VARIATION TIP: Add a little cooked ground beef or chicken to the tart for a more filling meal.

Per serving: Calories 527; Total fat 29g; Saturated fat 19g; Cholesterol 4mg; Carbs 60g; Fiber 15g; Protein 8g; Sodium 493mg

MUSHROOM AND PESTO CAULIFLOWER PIZZA

FATIGUE-FRIENDLY | BONE BOOSTER

Cauliflower and its magical shape-shifting abilities have put pizza back on the menu. This delicious pesto pizza is a healthy alternative to the typical red sauce and is topped simply with mushrooms and onion.

SERVES 2

Prep time: 10 minutes

Cook time: 30 minutes

1 cauliflower head, riced

⅓ cup arrowroot powder

1 teaspoon garlic powder

1 teaspoon onion powder

2 tablespoons dried oregano

1 tablespoon extra-virgin olive oil

Sea salt

¼ cup Nut-Free Basil Pesto (page 164)

1½ cups sliced mushrooms

¼ cup thinly sliced red onion

1. Preheat the oven to 350°F. Line a baking sheet with parchment paper.

2. In a microwave-safe dish, cook the cauliflower, partially covered, for 5 minutes on high in the microwave. Remove the dish and transfer the cauliflower to a clean dishtowel to cool. Once cool, tightly wrap the cauliflower in the towel and wring out as much moisture as possible.

3. In a large bowl, combine the cauliflower, arrowroot, garlic powder, onion powder, oregano, and olive oil. Season with salt. Mix well.

4. On the prepared baking sheet, shape the cauliflower mixture into a round disc and spread into a thin layer. Bake for 15 minutes.

5. Spread the pesto on the pizza, add the mushrooms, and top with the onion. Cook for an additional 10 minutes.

SUBSTITUTION TIP: You can use the Tomato-Free Marinara Sauce (page 165) in place of the pesto sauce, if desired.

Per serving: Calories 323; Total fat 14g; Saturated fat 3g; Cholesterol 8mg; Carbs 44g; Fiber 11g; Protein 11g; Sodium 399mg

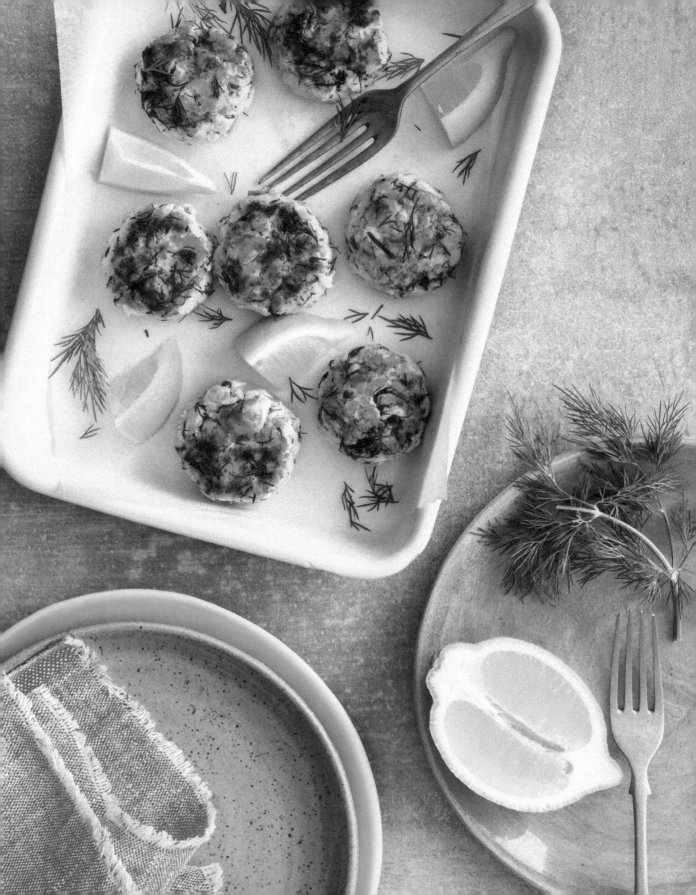

6 Fish and Seafood

CRISPY TUNA CAKES

FLARE SOOTHER | FATIGUE-FRIENDLY | CARDIO CARE | BONE BOOSTER

Without eggs, it can be hard to get cakes and patties to bind. But sweet potatoes are the right ingredient for the job. Paired with just a little gelatin to add extra firmness, these cakes are crisp and flavorful. Use a leftover baked sweet potato or quickly cook one in the microwave before beginning this recipe. Try canned salmon in place of the tuna for an easy switch that will produce equally delicious results with a whole different flavor.

SERVES 4

Prep time: 10 minutes

Cook time: 20 minutes

1 small baked sweet potato

2 (6-ounce) cans white tuna packed in water, drained

3 tablespoons coconut flour

2 garlic cloves, minced

1 tablespoon chopped fresh parsley

1 tablespoon unflavored gelatin

¼ cup warm water

1. Preheat the oven to 400°F. Line a baking sheet with parchment paper.

2. Remove the skin from the sweet potato, place the flesh in a large mixing bowl, and discard the skin. Add the tuna, coconut flour, garlic, and parsley.

3. In a small bowl, combine the gelatin and warm water and stir until the gelatin is completely dissolved. Let sit for 2 to 3 minutes until the water is absorbed. Stir the mixture into the tuna. Form into 12 small balls and press the balls into patties.

4. Arrange on a baking sheet in a single layer. Bake for 20 minutes.

COOKING TIP: To cook a sweet potato in the microwave, pierce its skin a couple of times with a fork, wrap it in a damp paper towel, and place it on a small plate. Cook for 5 minutes at high power and check for doneness. Cook for 3 to 4 minutes more, depending on the power of your microwave, until tender.

Per serving: Calories 302; Total fat 3g; Saturated fat 1g; Cholesterol 90mg; Carbs 17g; Fiber 5g; Protein 52g; Sodium 758mg

TUNA MUSHROOM MELTS

| FLARE SOOTHER | FATIGUE-FRIENDLY | CARDIO CARE | BONE BOOSTER |

Mushrooms have an undeniably meaty flavor, and here they help create an open-face sandwich that is filling and loaded with healthy fats and omega-3s.

SERVES 4

Prep time: 5 minutes

Cook time: 15 minutes

4 portabella mushroom caps, stemmed

1 tablespoon melted coconut oil

Sea salt

2 (6-ounce) cans white tuna packed in water, drained

1 avocado, chopped

1 celery stalk, finely chopped

½ onion, finely chopped

1. Preheat the oven to 375°F.

2. Brush the mushrooms with the coconut oil on both sides and season lightly with salt. Place gill-side up on a baking sheet and bake for 5 minutes.

3. While the mushrooms are cooking, in a medium bowl, mix the tuna, avocado, celery, and onion, and season with salt. Spoon the mixture into the mushroom caps and press it down into the caps.

4. Bake for 10 minutes until the tuna is heated through. Turn the broiler on and cook for 1 more minute until browned.

VARIATION TIP: This dish can be made as finger food using smaller brown mushroom caps, for a light snack or appetizer.

Per serving: Calories 328; Total fat 12g; Saturated fat 4g; Cholesterol 90mg; Carbs 6g; Fiber 3g; Protein 50g; Sodium 819mg

SEARED AHI TUNA WITH CHIMICHURRI

FLARE SOOTHER | FATIGUE-FRIENDLY | CARDIO CARE | BONE BOOSTER

Ahi tuna takes on whatever flavors you give it, and here the bold taste of chimichurri sauce brightens it exceptionally well. Make the chimichurri the night before, quickly sear the tuna, and you can have a meal on the table in fewer than 20 minutes.

SERVES 4

Prep time: 10 minutes

Cook time: 5 minutes

4 (6-ounce) ahi tuna steaks

½ teaspoon chopped fresh thyme

Sea salt

1 tablespoon extra-virgin olive oil

8 cups packed baby salad greens

1 recipe Chimichurri Sauce (page 163)

1. Season the tuna with the thyme and salt.

2. In a large skillet, heat the olive oil over high heat. Cook the tuna steaks for 2 minutes on each side, flipping once, until they are browned on the outside but still rare inside.

3. Serve the tuna on a bed of greens, topped with chimichurri sauce.

VARIATION TIP: The bitter notes of arugula are delicious in this salad. If your salad-greens blend doesn't include arugula, substitute packed baby arugula for up to half of the salad greens.

Per serving: Calories 406; Total fat 22g; Saturated fat 3g; Cholesterol 84mg; Carbs 8g; Fiber 2g; Protein 44g; Sodium 321mg

CRISPY TILAPIA STRIPS

FLARE SOOTHER	FATIGUE-FRIENDLY	KIDNEY SUPPORT	CARDIO CARE	BONE BOOSTER

Make this healthier version of crispy breaded fish sticks that skips the wheat-based breading and instead is loaded with coconut flavor. Pair it with Cabbage and Bacon Slaw (page 72).

SERVES 4

Prep time: 10 minutes

Cook time: 10 minutes

1 pound tilapia fillets, cut lengthwise into strips

Sea salt

¼ teaspoon garlic powder

¼ teaspoon onion powder

½ cup coconut flour

¼ cup coconut oil

1. Season the fish with salt, garlic powder, and onion powder.

2. Place the coconut flour on a flat plate and roll the fillets in it, pressing firmly so the flour sticks.

3. In a deep skillet, heat the coconut oil over medium-high heat. Slowly add the fish to the hot oil and cook for 3 to 4 minutes on each side, carefully flipping once, until well browned.

COOKING TIP: Be patient and wait until the breading is a deep golden brown before flipping the fish. Use a firm spatula to gently flip the pieces without breaking off the breading.

Per serving: Calories 332; Total fat 18g; Saturated fat 14g; Cholesterol 55mg; Carbs 20g; Fiber 12g; Protein 25g; Sodium 99mg

EASY MACKEREL

| FLARE SOOTHER | FATIGUE-FRIENDLY | KIDNEY SUPPORT | CARDIO CARE | BONE BOOSTER |

Mackerel is a fatty fish that's loaded with omega-3 fatty acids and is often sold at a fraction of the price of other equally fatty fishes, such as salmon. It has a mild flavor and is easy to cook. One of the simplest preparations is the one below, using just salt and olive oil to create a fabulous cooked fish.

SERVES 4

Prep time: 5 minutes, plus 15 minutes to marinate

Cook time: 10 minutes

2 tablespoons melted coconut oil, divided

4 (6-ounce) mackerel fillets, with skin

2 teaspoons sea salt

2 garlic cloves, sliced

1. In a medium bowl, rub 1 tablespoon of the coconut oil on both sides of the mackerel. Sprinkle with the salt on both sides and let the fish rest at room temperature for 15 minutes.

2. In a large skillet, heat the remaining 1 tablespoon of coconut oil over medium-high heat. Scatter the garlic in the pan and immediately add the fish, skin-side down. Cook the fish for 5 to 6 minutes. When the flesh is almost completely white and cooked through, flip the fillets and cook for 1 minute more.

COOKING TIP: Mackerel is a thin fish, weighing typically a little over a pound per fish. Because it cooks quickly, don't walk away from the stove, and be ready to flip it earlier if the flesh turns from translucent to opaque quicker than the cooking time given here.

Per serving: Calories 291; Total fat 23g; Saturated fat 10g; Cholesterol 66mg; Carbs 1g; Fiber 0g; Protein 21g; Sodium 809mg

HERBED HALIBUT IN PARCHMENT

FLARE SOOTHER | FATIGUE-FRIENDLY | CARDIO CARE | BONE BOOSTER

Parchment-paper packets are the perfect way to cook tender and juicy fish. These simple packets are loaded with fresh herb flavor and come alive with just a bit of salt and lemon. Because the packets are sealed, the fish stays tender and your job of cooking is pretty much done when they go in the oven.

SERVES 2

Prep time: 5 minutes

Cook time: 20 minutes

2 (6-ounce) halibut fillets

4 scallions, cut into 3-inch segments

1¼ cups sliced brown mushrooms

2 garlic cloves, minced

1 tablespoon extra-virgin olive oil

Sea salt

1 lemon, sliced

1 tablespoon chopped fresh basil

1 tablespoon chopped fresh chives

1. Preheat the oven to 375°F.

2. Tear off two pieces of parchment paper, each about 12 inches long. On each piece of paper, place half of the scallions, half of the mushrooms, and half of the garlic. Place a halibut fillet on top of each portion of vegetables. Drizzle the fillets with the olive oil and season with salt. Place two or three lemon slices on top of each fillet. Sprinkle the basil and chives on top.

3. Fold the parchment paper over the top of the fish and bring the edges together. Then make several small folds around the edges to seal the packets. Arrange the packets in a single layer on a baking sheet.

4. Bake for 15 to 18 minutes until the fish is cooked through and flakes easily. Be careful when opening the packets, as steam will escape.

SUBSTITUTION TIP: Use any other favorite firm fish in these packets. If you don't have parchment, aluminum foil will also work.

Per serving: Calories 232; Total fat 10g; Saturated fat 2g; Cholesterol 45mg; Carbs 5g; Fiber 1g; Protein 31g; Sodium 201mg

ITALIAN POACHED SEA BASS

| FLARE SOOTHER | FATIGUE-FRIENDLY | KIDNEY SUPPORT | CARDIO CARE | BONE BOOSTER |

Poaching is another simple method for cooking fish that produces flavorful, tender results with minimal work. The delicate flavor of sea bass pairs well with basil and olives in this quick dish. Serve it with Turnip "Rice" (page 51) for a light meal.

SERVES 4

Prep time: 5 minutes

Cook time: 10 minutes

1 tablespoon extra-virgin olive oil

1 small red onion, cut into thin wedges

4 garlic cloves, sliced

½ teaspoon sea salt, divided

1 cup water

4 (4-ounce) skinless sea bass fillets

½ cup pitted Kalamata olives

¼ cup chopped fresh parsley

3 tablespoons chopped fresh basil

1. In a large skillet, heat the olive oil over medium heat. Add the onion, garlic, and ¼ teaspoon of the salt, and cook for 3 to 5 minutes until softened.

2. Add the water and bring to a simmer. Meanwhile, season the fish with the remaining ¼ teaspoon of salt.

3. Carefully slide the fish into the simmering liquid, cover, and cook for 10 minutes until the fish is cooked through and easily flakes with a fork. Add the olives to heat through.

4. Using a slotted spoon, transfer the fish, olives, and onion to a serving plate. Serve, garnished with the parsley and basil.

SUBSTITUTION TIP: Substitute snapper, cod, or grouper for the sea bass.

Per serving: Calories 254; Total fat 15g; Saturated fat 3g; Cholesterol 0mg; Carbs 4g; Fiber 2g; Protein 26g; Sodium 361mg

GARLIC-BASIL MAHI MAHI

| FLARE SOOTHER | FATIGUE-FRIENDLY | KIDNEY SUPPORT | CARDIO CARE | BONE BOOSTER |

Mahi mahi is a firm fish with a mild flavor, making it a popular choice for people who are not big fans of fish. In this quick-prep recipe, it is seasoned with garlic, lemon, and basil.

SERVES 4

Prep time: 5 minutes

Cook time: 10 minutes

2 tablespoons melted coconut oil, divided

Juice of 1 lemon

2 garlic cloves, minced

½ teaspoon sea salt, divided

2 tablespoons chopped fresh basil leaves

4 (6-ounce) mahi mahi fillets

1. In a small bowl, combine 1 tablespoon of the coconut oil, the lemon juice, the garlic, ¼ teaspoon of the salt, and the basil. Set the sauce aside.

2. In a large skillet, heat the remaining 1 tablespoon of coconut oil over medium-high heat. Season the fish with the remaining ¼ teaspoon of salt.

3. Cook the fillets for 3 to 5 minutes per side, flipping once, until the fish flakes and is opaque. Remove the fillets to serving plates.

4. Add the sauce to the skillet and heat for 1 minute over medium heat. Spoon the sauce over the fillets and serve.

COOKING TIP: With a firm fish such as mahi mahi, aim for a nicely uniform browned exterior before flipping. Make sure the oil is hot before adding the fish to the pan and be sure to use a metal spatula to help prevent any sticking.

Per serving: Calories 196; Total fat 7g; Saturated fat 6g; Cholesterol 60mg; Carbs 1g; Fiber 0g; Protein 32g; Sodium 377mg

BAKED SALMON STEAKS

FLARE SOOTHER	FATIGUE-FRIENDLY	KIDNEY SUPPORT	CARDIO CARE	BONE BOOSTER

Salmon steaks are easy to make, fun to eat, and somehow seem meatier than fillets. This simple dish takes just minutes to put together and leaves you with enough time to make a simple side dish. Or better yet, roast some vegetables along with the salmon and your meal will cook while you unwind from your day.

SERVES 2

Prep time: 5 minutes

Cook time: 20 minutes

2 (6- to 8-ounce) salmon steaks

1 tablespoon extra-virgin olive oil

Juice of 1 lemon

1 tablespoon minced fresh parsley

½ teaspoon dried thyme

Sea salt

1. Preheat the oven to 400°F.

2. Place the salmon in a baking dish. Drizzle the olive oil and lemon juice over the fish. Sprinkle the parsley and thyme over the top and season lightly with salt.

3. Bake for 15 to 20 minutes until the salmon flakes with a fork.

VARIATION TIP: Use a different combination of herbs to make something a little different. Tarragon and basil are two that complement salmon well.

Per serving: Calories 444; Total fat 27g; Saturated fat 5g; Cholesterol 137mg; Carbs 1g; Fiber 0g; Protein 47g; Sodium 227mg

TURMERIC COCONUT SALMON

FLARE SOOTHER | FATIGUE-FRIENDLY | KIDNEY SUPPORT | CARDIO CARE | BONE BOOSTER

Turmeric is a natural anti-inflammatory, and when mixed with luxurious coconut milk, it makes a wonderful base of flavor for salmon. Turmeric contains one of the highest levels of beta-carotene, is a powerful antioxidant, and has a unique astringent flavor that is highlighted well in this dish.

SERVES 2

Prep time: 5 minutes

Cook time: 10 minutes

3 garlic cloves, minced

½ teaspoon ground turmeric

¼ teaspoon sea salt

1 tablespoon coconut oil

½ pound boneless salmon fillet, skin on

½ cup full-fat coconut milk

1. In a small bowl, mix the garlic, turmeric, and salt. Set aside.

2. In a large skillet, heat the coconut oil over medium-high heat. Spread the turmeric-garlic mixture over the flesh side of the fish. When the oil is hot, place the fish in the skillet, skin-side up, and cook for 2 to 3 minutes until browned. Flip and continue to cook on the skin side for 3 more minutes.

3. Pour the coconut milk over the fish, lifting it gently with the spatula to get some of the coconut milk under the fish. Spoon the sauce over the salmon, cover, reduce the heat to medium-low, and cook for 2 to 4 more minutes until cooked through.

SUBSTITUTION TIP: Halibut also works well in this recipe.

Per serving: Calories 315; Total fat 23g; Saturated fat 19g; Cholesterol 55mg; Carbs 5g; Fiber 3g; Protein 25g; Sodium 484mg

LEMON-HERBED SALMON CAKES

| FLARE SOOTHER | FATIGUE-FRIENDLY | KIDNEY SUPPORT | CARDIO CARE | BONE BOOSTER |

Salmon cakes are a versatile and simple dish easily made with leftover salmon. Or, in a pinch, you can use canned to make the whole thing even easier. If you do use canned, look for boneless, skinless canned salmon, and be sure to drain it well so your patties are not soggy.

SERVES 4

Prep time: 5 minutes

Cook time: 20 minutes

10 ounces cooked salmon (canned or cooked and crumbled fillets)

1 scallion, thinly sliced

1 tablespoon chopped fresh dill

Juice and zest of 1 lemon

¼ cup coconut flour

2 tablespoons coconut oil, softened

Sea salt

1. Preheat the oven to 400°F. Line a baking sheet with parchment paper.

2. In a mixing bowl, combine the salmon, scallion, dill, lemon juice and zest, coconut flour, and coconut oil. Season with salt. Mix well.

3. Form the mixture into six small patties and place on the prepared baking sheet. Bake for 20 minutes until lightly browned. Let rest for 5 minutes before serving.

VARIATION TIP: Serve the salmon on a lightly dressed bed of greens for a complete meal, or pair them with a vegetable side dish or two, if you have a little more time.

Per serving: Calories 216; Total fat 13g; Saturated fat 8g; Cholesterol 31mg; Carbs 11g; Fiber 6g; Protein 16g; Sodium 92mg

SWEET POTATO CRAB CAKES

FLARE SOOTHER | FATIGUE-FRIENDLY | CARDIO CARE

There's no need to use an egg for binding when a sweet potato does the same job. Here, it also adds a hint of sweetness to this otherwise savory cake. Use a leftover baked sweet potato or cook one in the microwave (be sure to pierce the sweet potato with a fork and wrap it in a paper towel) for 5 to 7 minutes until soft.

SERVES 2

Prep time: 5 minutes

Cook time: 10 minutes

1 (6-ounce) can lump crabmeat

1 cup cooked sweet potato

¼ cup arrowroot powder

2 tablespoons chopped fresh parsley

Juice of ½ lemon

¼ teaspoon sea salt

1 tablespoon extra-virgin olive oil

1. In a medium bowl, combine the crabmeat, sweet potato, arrowroot, parsley, lemon juice, and salt. Shape the mixture into four patties.

2. In a large skillet, heat the olive oil over medium heat. Cook the patties on each side for 3 to 4 minutes until browned, flipping once.

INGREDIENT TIP: Look for canned lump crabmeat in the canned-foods section of the grocery store, near the tuna. Alternatively, if it's available, you can use packaged lump crabmeat found in the fish or deli section.

Per serving: Calories 286; Total fat 14g; Saturated fat 1g; Cholesterol 48mg; Carbs 39g; Fiber 5g; Protein 15g; Sodium 755mg

ZUCCHINI NOODLES IN CLAM SAUCE

FLARE SOOTHER	FATIGUE-FRIENDLY	KIDNEY SUPPORT	CARDIO CARE	BONE BOOSTER

There are so many ways you can prepare zucchini noodles, and this is another great method you'll love. It is quick to make and features plenty of good fats and omega-3 fatty acids that your body needs. Use shelled frozen clam meat, to minimize your prep time in the kitchen and give your hands a break.

SERVES 4

Prep time: 10 minutes

Cook time: 10 minutes

2 tablespoons extra-virgin olive oil

3 garlic cloves, minced

1 pound frozen clam meat, thawed and chopped

½ cup full-fat coconut milk

¼ cup chopped parsley

Sea salt

2 zucchini, spiralized or cut into thin noodle-size strips

1. In a large skillet, heat the olive oil over medium heat. Add the garlic and cook for 30 seconds until fragrant.

2. Add the clam meat, mix well, and cook for 4 to 5 minutes, stirring regularly, until cooked through. Add the coconut milk and bring to a simmer. Reduce the heat to medium-low. Add the parsley and season with salt.

3. Add the zucchini noodles and cook for 1 to 2 minutes until softened.

SUBSTITUTION TIP: If you can't find frozen clam meat, substitute canned instead. Be sure to rinse and drain it well.

Per serving: Calories 466; Total fat 31g; Saturated fat 15g; Cholesterol 77mg; Carbs 18g; Fiber 4g; Protein 33g; Sodium 277mg

MUSSELS IN WHITE WINE SAUCE

| FLARE SOOTHER | FATIGUE-FRIENDLY | KIDNEY SUPPORT | CARDIO CARE | BONE BOOSTER |

Mussels are a great source of vitamin B$_{12}$, iron, zinc, and selenium; are loaded with protein; and are quick-cooking, making them a perfect dinner choice. This dish is great served over a bed of lightly cooked zucchini or squash noodles.

SERVES 4

Prep time: 5 minutes

Cook time: 15 minutes

2 tablespoons coconut oil

½ small onion, minced

1 cup dry white wine or bone broth

2 fresh parsley sprigs

2 fresh thyme sprigs

2 pounds fresh cleaned mussels

Sea salt

Juice of ½ lemon

Chopped fresh parsley, for garnish

1. In a large skillet, heat the coconut oil over medium-high heat. Cook the onion for 3 to 5 minutes until tender.

2. Add the wine, parsley, and thyme, and bring to a boil. Reduce the heat and simmer for 3 to 4 minutes, reducing the sauce and cooking the alcohol from it.

3. Add the mussels, cover, and cook for 4 minutes, shaking the skillet a couple of times while the mussels cook.

4. Open the skillet after 4 minutes and check to see if the shells have opened. If they have, they are done. If not, cook another minute and check again. Discard any unopened shells.

5. Season with salt and the lemon juice. Serve the mussels in bowls with the wine sauce, garnished with parsley.

INGREDIENT TIP: Before cooking, place the mussels in a bath of ice water and scrub them with a brush to remove dirt and sand. Remove the beard (the small, rough patch hanging out of the shell) from each mussel by pulling firmly on it with your hand or a dishtowel. Discard any mussels that are opened before cooking.

Per serving: Calories 307; Total fat 12g; Saturated fat 7g; Cholesterol 63mg; Carbs 11g; Fiber 0g; Protein 27g; Sodium 711mg

LEMONY SHRIMP ZUCCHINI NOODLES

FLARE SOOTHER | **FATIGUE-FRIENDLY** | **KIDNEY SUPPORT**

If you have a hard time giving up flavorful noodles, this is a dish to try. While zucchini noodles are not a perfect replacement for the wheat variety, they do satisfy a noodle craving without bloating you with starchy carbs. Zucchini noodles hold sauce well and are perfect in this light summer dish, which will fill you up without the discomfort of wheat.

SERVES 4

Prep time: 15 minutes

Cook time: 8 minutes

2 tablespoons extra-virgin olive oil

1 pound shrimp, peeled and deveined

3 garlic cloves, minced

1 cup thinly sliced snow peas

2 medium zucchini, spiralized or cut into thin noodle-size strips

Juice of 1 lemon

Sea salt

½ cup chopped fresh parsley

1. In a large skillet, heat the olive oil over medium heat. Add the shrimp and cook for 2 to 3 minutes, stirring regularly, until they're pink and opaque. Remove from the skillet and set aside.

2. In the same skillet, cook the garlic for 30 seconds until fragrant. Add the peas and cook for 2 minutes, stirring, until softened.

3. Add the zucchini noodles and cook for 2 more minutes. Return the shrimp to the skillet and drizzle with the lemon juice. Season with salt and garnish with the parsley.

VARIATION TIP: Add 1 cup of thinly sliced chicken breast (reduce the shrimp to ½ pound) before you add the shrimp, and cook until browned for a chicken-and-shrimp noodle combination.

Per serving: Calories 192; Total fat 8g; Saturated fat 1g; Cholesterol 180mg; Carbs 7g; Fiber 2g; Protein 25g; Sodium 206mg

SHRIMP TACOS WITH PINEAPPLE-AVOCADO SALSA

FLARE SOOTHER | FATIGUE-FRIENDLY

Green plantains create the tortillas here, and they couldn't be easier to make. The ingredient list may look long, but if you break it down into the three elements—salsa, tortillas, and shrimp—it is super manageable and easy to pull together without too much work.

SERVES 4 (2 TACOS EACH)

Prep time: 10 minutes
Cook time: 30 minutes

FOR THE TORTILLAS

2 large green plantains, peeled and coarsely chopped

¼ cup coconut oil

1 teaspoon sea salt

FOR THE SALSA

1 (14-ounce) can pineapple chunks, drained

1 avocado, peeled, seeded, and chopped

2 tablespoons freshly squeezed lime juice

1 tablespoon extra-virgin olive oil

¼ cup chopped red onion

Sea salt

FOR THE SHRIMP

1 pound shrimp, peeled and deveined

Sea salt

1 tablespoon extra-virgin olive oil

TO MAKE THE TORTILLAS

1. Preheat the oven to 400°F. Line two baking sheets with parchment paper.

2. In a food processor, combine the plantains, coconut oil, and salt. Process until smooth.

3. Spread the mixture on the prepared baking sheets in four circles for each sheet, each about 4 or 5 inches in diameter and about ¼ inch thick. Bake for 20 to 30 minutes until golden brown and cooked through.

4. Let cool for about 10 minutes before serving, flipping once to allow the bottoms to cool.

TO MAKE THE SALSA

In a medium bowl, combine the pineapple, avocado, lime juice, olive oil, and onion. Season with salt.

TO MAKE THE SHRIMP

1. Season the shrimp lightly with salt.

2. In a large skillet, heat the olive oil over medium heat. Add the shrimp and cook for 3 to 5 minutes, stirring frequently, until just cooked through and opaque.

3. Serve the shrimp in the tortillas, topped with the salsa.

COOKING TIP: Plantain tortillas work great for tacos, but they taste best when still warm. If needed, make the salsa and shrimp the night before, then mix up the batter and make the tortillas right before serving.

Per serving: Calories 440; Total fat 29g; Saturated fat 14g; Cholesterol 239mg; Carbs 48g; Fiber 7g; Protein 33g; Sodium 649mg

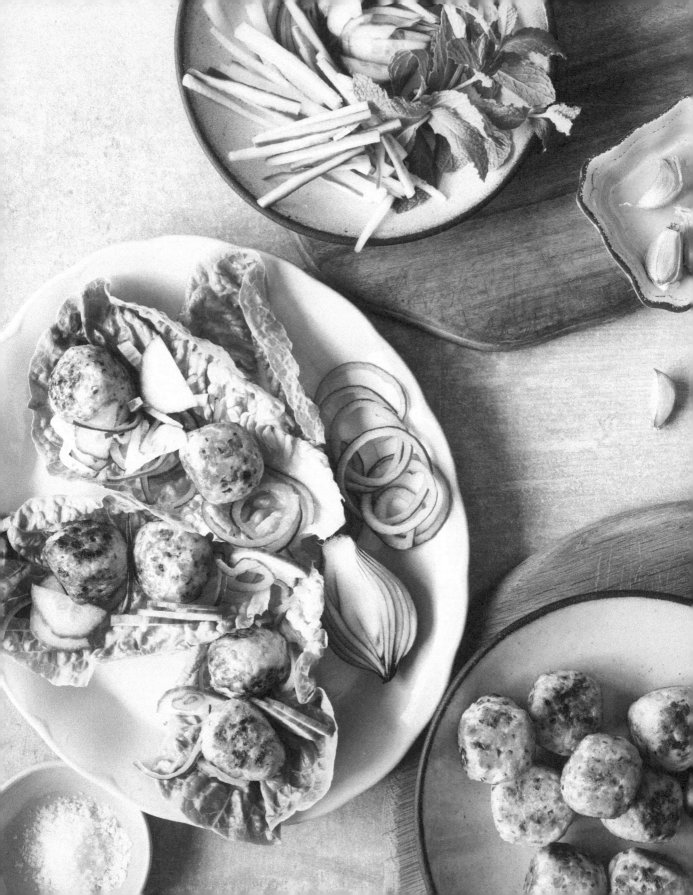

7 Poultry and Meat

CHICKEN SALAD WITH APPLE AND GRAPES

FLARE SOOTHER | FATIGUE-FRIENDLY | KIDNEY SUPPORT

Chicken salad is a wonderful dish for busy days. With its apple and grapes, this salad packs in plenty of vitamins. Serve the chicken as a salad, as in this recipe, or make it into sandwich wraps with either leaf lettuce or Plantain Wraps (page 46).

SERVES 4

Prep time: 10 minutes

2 cups chopped
cooked chicken

1 celery stalk, finely chopped

2 scallions, thinly sliced

1 small Granny Smith apple,
cored and finely chopped

½ cup red seedless grapes

1 recipe Creamy Egg-Free
Mayo (page 154)

Sea salt

8 cups mixed baby
salad greens

1. In a large bowl, toss the chicken, celery, scallions, apple, grapes, and mayo. Mix well and season with salt.

2. Divide the salad greens among four plates and serve the chicken salad over the greens.

VARIATION TIP: Instead of serving on a bed of greens, cut a cucumber lengthwise and remove its seeds. Scoop the chicken salad into half of the cucumber and top with the remaining cucumber half. Cut in half crosswise and serve as a sandwich.

Per serving: Calories 359; Total fat 22g; Saturated fat 9g; Cholesterol 54mg; Carbs 21g; Fiber 4g; Protein 24g; Sodium 355mg

COCONUT CHICKEN STRIPS

FATIGUE-FRIENDLY | KIDNEY SUPPORT

Chicken strips aren't just for kids. These tasty pieces of chicken breast are rolled in coconut flour, making them wonderfully flavorful, gluten-free, and crisp, yet without all the fat from frying. To make ahead, you can prep the strips through step 3, freeze them flat on a baking sheet, and when frozen, pack into a zip-top freezer bag and freeze for up to 1 month. Add 5 to 7 minutes to the baking time if you're cooking them from frozen.

SERVES 4

Prep time: 5 minutes

Cook time: 15 minutes

½ cup coconut flour

½ teaspoon sea salt

1 teaspoon dried Italian seasoning mix

¼ cup coconut oil, melted

1 pound boneless, skinless chicken breast, cut lengthwise into 1½-inch strips

1. Preheat the oven to 400°F. Line a baking sheet with parchment paper.

2. In a small bowl, mix the coconut flour, sea salt, and Italian seasoning.

3. Pour the coconut oil into another small bowl. Coat each chicken strip in coconut oil, shake it over the bowl to remove any excess, and roll it in the coconut flour mixture. Place the chicken strips in a single layer on the prepared baking sheet.

4. Bake for 6 to 8 minutes, flip, and bake for 6 to 8 minutes more until browned and the juices run clear.

VARIATION TIP: For a juicier piece of chicken, use boneless, skinless thighs instead. Be sure to trim the thigh of excess fat and cut each thigh into 2 or 3 pieces. Follow the recipe as written.

Per serving: Calories 367; Total fat 20g; Saturated fat 14g; Cholesterol 73mg; Carbs 20g; Fiber 12g; Protein 28g; Sodium 272mg

GLAZED STICKY WINGS

FATIGUE-FRIENDLY | KIDNEY SUPPORT

Sticky wings are always a crowd pleaser, and there is no need to give them up. The honey adds the desirable sticky, sweet element to the wings and coconut aminos brings the savory umami flavor that is so important for preparing great wings.

SERVES 6

Prep time: 5 minutes, plus 1 hour to marinate

Cook time: 45 minutes

¼ cup honey

¼ cup freshly squeezed lemon juice

2 tablespoons coconut aminos

2 tablespoons apple cider vinegar

2 teaspoons garlic powder

⅓ cup water

3 pounds chicken wings, split, tips discarded

Coconut oil, for greasing

1. In a small saucepan over medium heat, mix the honey, lemon juice, coconut aminos, vinegar, garlic powder, and water. Bring to a simmer and cook for 3 minutes until slightly thickened. Let cool.

2. In a medium bowl or plastic bag, mix the marinade with the wings. Cover and refrigerate for at least 1 hour or as long as overnight.

3. Preheat the oven to 400°F. Grease a large baking dish with coconut oil.

4. Arrange the chicken wings in a single layer in the baking dish. Cook for 45 minutes, flipping once about halfway through, until cooked through.

VARIATION TIP: To make hot wings without using hot peppers (which are nightshades), add 2 tablespoons or more of horseradish to the marinade.

Per serving: Calories 555; Total fat 36g; Saturated fat 10g; Cholesterol 170mg; Carbs 14g; Fiber 0g; Protein 42g; Sodium 179mg

HERB-ROASTED CHICKEN LEGS

FATIGUE-FRIENDLY | **KIDNEY SUPPORT**

Chicken legs are a very easy main dish that is delicious and requires minimal effort. Because they are a darker cut of meat, they remain tender and always turn out great. This herb combination of thyme and oregano is a warming blend that pairs well with just about any side dish you can make.

SERVES 6

Prep time: 5 minutes

Cook time: 35 minutes

6 chicken legs

1 tablespoon avocado oil

3 fresh thyme sprigs, leaves removed and chopped

1 teaspoon garlic powder

1 teaspoon dried oregano

½ teaspoon sea salt

Juice of 1 lemon

1. Preheat the oven to 425°F.

2. In a medium bowl, toss the chicken with the avocado oil to coat. Sprinkle the thyme, garlic powder, oregano, and salt over the chicken and stir to coat.

3. Arrange the chicken in a single layer in a baking dish and squeeze the lemon juice over the top. Bake for 20 minutes, then lower the oven temperature to 350°F and cook for 15 minutes more, until the juices run clear.

SUBSTITUTION TIP: This recipe also works great with chicken thighs or a combination of legs and thighs.

Per serving: Calories 303; Total fat 21g; Saturated fat 6g; Cholesterol 127mg; Carbs 1g; Fiber 0g; Protein 28g; Sodium 276mg

LEMON-OLIVE CHICKEN PROVENCAL

FLARE SOOTHER | FATIGUE-FRIENDLY | BONE BOOSTER

If you like the salty, briny flavor of olives, this simple dish is going to excite you. Pair it with some sautéed green beans or serve it over Turnip "Rice" (page 51) for an easy meal. Chicken thighs are often fatty, so be sure to trim them well before cooking.

SERVES 4

Prep time: 5 minutes

Cook time: 30 minutes

1 onion, chopped

4 to 6 boneless, skinless chicken thighs

¼ teaspoon sea salt

1 lemon, thinly sliced and seeded

1 teaspoon chopped fresh rosemary

½ cup pitted green olives

½ cup Chicken Bone Broth (page 151)

¼ cup chopped fresh parsley

1. Preheat the oven to 375°F.

2. In a medium baking dish, sprinkle the onion on the bottom. Season the chicken with salt and arrange the thighs on top of the onion. Place the lemon slices on top of the thighs and sprinkle with the rosemary.

3. Add the olives and bone broth to the dish and cover the pan tightly with aluminum foil. Bake for 30 minutes until cooked through. Serve garnished with the parsley.

SUBSTITUTION TIP: Kalamata olives also work well in this recipe.

Per serving: Calories 220; Total fat 8g; Saturated fat 2g; Cholesterol 143mg; Carbs 4g; Fiber 1g; Protein 34g; Sodium 398mg

GARLIC-MINT CHICKEN MEATBALL WRAPS

FLARE SOOTHER | FATIGUE-FRIENDLY | KIDNEY SUPPORT

Mint is a highly versatile herb that can be used for both sweet and savory dishes with great results. It lends a wonderful flavor to the chicken in these meatballs—a cooling herb that complements the lettuce wrap it is served in.

SERVES 4

Prep time: 10 minutes

Cook time: 15 minutes

1 pound ground chicken

2 tablespoons fish sauce

1 onion, finely chopped

3 garlic cloves, minced

2 tablespoons chopped fresh mint

1 tablespoon chopped fresh cilantro

½ teaspoon sea salt

1 head leaf lettuce

1 cucumber, halved lengthwise and thinly sliced

1 small red onion, halved and sliced

1. Preheat the oven to 400°F. Line a baking sheet with parchment paper.

2. In a large bowl, combine the chicken, fish sauce, onion, garlic, mint, cilantro, and salt. Mix well and shape into 1½-inch balls. Arrange on the prepared baking sheet.

3. Cook for 15 minutes until browned and cooked through.

4. Serve the meatballs in lettuce leaf wraps, garnished with the cucumber and onion.

VARIATION TIP: These also go great with the Plantain Wraps (page 46). Get the wraps cooking first, before you make the meatballs, and they will be ready to go right around the same time.

Per serving: Calories 209; Total fat 9g; Saturated fat 3g; Cholesterol 96mg; Carbs 9g; Fiber 3g; Protein 23g; Sodium 1044mg

ITALIAN-SEASONED CHICKEN SKEWERS

FLARE SOOTHER | **FATIGUE-FRIENDLY**

Marinating chicken and vegetables in a simple herb-infused vinaigrette is so easy and adds so much flavor. Try to marinate the dish for at least an hour, but if you are in a rush, even 30 minutes will produce flavorful results. Your oven's broil setting makes these skewers possible all year long no matter where you live, but if you can, try cooking them on your barbecue grill.

SERVES 4

Prep time: 5 minutes,
plus 1 hour to marinate

Cook time: 15 minutes

¼ cup extra-virgin olive oil

2 tablespoons white
wine vinegar

2 tablespoons freshly
squeezed lemon juice

3 garlic cloves, minced

1 teaspoon dried basil

¼ teaspoon dried oregano

¼ teaspoon sea salt

1 pound boneless, skinless
chicken breast, cut into
1-inch cubes

1 small zucchini, cut into
2-inch cubes

1 small yellow summer
squash, cut into 2-inch cubes

1 cup small mushrooms

1 red onion, cut into wedges

8 cups mixed salad greens

1. Preheat a grill or your broiler.

2. In a small bowl, combine the olive oil, vinegar, lemon juice, garlic, basil, oregano, and salt.

3. Thread the chicken and vegetables onto skewers, alternating the items. Place all the skewers in a large baking dish or a zip-top bag. Pour the marinade over the skewers and marinate for about 1 hour.

4. Over a hot grill or on a rimmed baking sheet under the broiler, cook the kebabs for about 15 minutes total, flipping several times, until the chicken is cooked through and the vegetables are softened and lightly charred. Serve over the mixed salad greens.

COOKING TIP: You will need metal or wood skewers for this recipe. If you're using wood, soak them in water for 1 hour before you marinate the chicken.

Per serving: Calories 308; Total fat 16g; Saturated fat 2g; Cholesterol 73mg; Carbs 14g; Fiber 1g; Protein 29g; Sodium 254mg

ONE-SKILLET CHICKEN THIGHS AND ROOT VEGGIES

FLARE SOOTHER | CARDIO CARE | BONE BOOSTER

One-skillet dishes are some of the simplest ways to whip up a well-balanced meal. In this dish, rutabaga, sweet potato, and turnips all cook to tenderness, while the chicken thighs are juicy and loaded with flavor. The leftovers keep well, so eat this for a quick lunch throughout the week.

SERVES 4

Prep time: 5 minutes

Cook time: 40 minutes

2 tablespoons coconut oil

1 medium onion, chopped into ½-inch pieces

3 garlic cloves, minced

4 to 6 boneless, skinless chicken thighs

1 small sweet potato, chopped into ½-inch pieces

1 small rutabaga, chopped into ½-inch pieces

1 turnip, chopped into ½-inch pieces

½ cup Chicken Bone Broth (page 151) or water

½ teaspoon sea salt

2 fresh thyme sprigs, leaves removed and chopped

1. In a large skillet, heat the coconut oil over medium heat. Cook the onion and garlic for 2 to 3 minutes until slightly softened and fragrant. Add the chicken thighs and cook on each side for 2 to 3 minutes until browned.

2. Arrange the sweet potato, rutabaga, and turnip around the chicken and add the broth and salt. Bring to a boil, reduce the heat to low, cover, and simmer for 20 to 30 minutes until the chicken is cooked through and the vegetables are tender. Serve garnished with the thyme.

INGREDIENT TIP: If chopping hard vegetables is too difficult, look for precut vegetables in the chilled packaged food or produce section of the grocery store. While this exact combination of vegetables may not be available, there are often winter squash and other hard veggies precut for convenience that can be used in a skillet dish such as this.

Per serving: Calories 322; Total fat 14g; Saturated fat 7g; Cholesterol 143mg; Carbs 16g; Fiber 3g; Protein 35g; Sodium 433mg

SPICE-RUBBED ROASTED CHICKEN

FATIGUE-FRIENDLY | KIDNEY SUPPORT

Roasting a whole chicken allows you to create several meals from just one cooking session. Eat it first as a main course and then use the leftovers to make Homestyle Chicken and Vegetable Soup (page 81) and Chicken Salad with Apple and Grapes (page 116).

SERVES 8

Prep time: 5 minutes

Cook time: 1 hour

1 (3-pound) chicken

1 onion, quartered

3 fresh rosemary sprigs

4 fresh thyme sprigs

1 tablespoon coconut oil, melted

1 teaspoon sea salt

1 tablespoon garlic powder

1 tablespoon onion powder

1. Preheat the oven to 425°F.

2. Stuff the chicken cavity with the onion, rosemary, and thyme. Rub the chicken skin with the coconut oil and sprinkle evenly with the salt, garlic powder, and onion powder.

3. Place the chicken on a rack in a roasting pan and cook for 45 minutes to 1 hour until the chicken is cooked through and the juices run clear.

4. Let the chicken rest for 10 minutes before carving and serving.

SUBSTITUTION TIP: Use other fresh herbs that you have on hand for stuffing the chicken. Parsley, sage, and cilantro all pair well with chicken, and a few lemon slices are also a great addition.

Per serving: Calories 196; Total fat 10g; Saturated fat 4g; Cholesterol 83mg; Carbs 3g; Fiber 0g; Protein 23g; Sodium 309mg

HERB-CRUSTED PORK TENDERLOIN

FATIGUE-FRIENDLY | **KIDNEY SUPPORT**

Beef tenderloin may get all the fame, but a pork tenderloin can be just as great. Using fresh rosemary and thyme, this simple cut of meat comes alive in fewer than 30 minutes. Pair it with roasted vegetables that you can cook alongside the meat, and you are on your way to an easy and satisfying meal.

SERVES 4

Prep time: 5 minutes

Cook time: 30 minutes

1 (1-pound) boneless pork tenderloin

3 tablespoons coconut oil, melted, divided

1 fresh rosemary sprig, leaves removed and chopped

2 fresh thyme sprigs, leaves removed and chopped

3 garlic cloves, minced

1 teaspoon sea salt

1. Preheat the oven to 425°F.

2. Rub 2 tablespoons of the coconut oil all over the tenderloin.

3. In a small bowl, combine the rosemary, thyme, garlic, and salt. Rub this mixture onto the pork.

4. Heat an oven-safe skillet over medium-high heat and pour in the remaining 1 tablespoon of coconut oil. Sear the pork for about 2 minutes on all sides until browned. Transfer the skillet to the oven and cook for 15 to 20 minutes until cooked through and the meat registers 145°F on a meat thermometer. Tent with aluminum foil and let rest for 10 minutes. Slice and serve.

COOKING TIP: Letting meat rest after cooking allows the juices to redistribute, leaving you with a juicier cut of meat. Be sure to allow time for this, or all the meat's juices will spill out when it is cut.

Per serving: Calories 206; Total fat 13g; Saturated fat 10g; Cholesterol 60mg; Carbs 1g; Fiber 0g; Protein 22g; Sodium 798mg

SKIRT STEAK ON A BED OF GREENS

FATIGUE-FRIENDLY | KIDNEY SUPPORT

Skirt steak is perfect for topping a salad. It is a slightly fattier cut of beef, but when cooked just right, that fat renders beautifully and you are left with a juicy and flavorful masterpiece of a salad that is perfect as a main course, dressed with a lime vinaigrette. The dressing and greens are best mixed right before serving.

SERVES 6

Prep time: 5 minutes

Cook time: 10 minutes

1 (1½-pound) skirt steak

Sea salt

4 tablespoons freshly squeezed lime juice, divided

1 tablespoon coconut oil

1 shallot, minced

2 tablespoons extra-virgin olive oil

2 garlic cloves, minced

8 cups mixed baby greens

2 scallions, chopped

1. Season the steak with salt and 1 tablespoon of the lime juice.

2. In a large skillet, heat the coconut oil over medium-high heat. Cook the steak for 4 to 5 minutes, flip, and cook 4 to 5 minutes more. Remove from the skillet, tent with a piece of aluminum foil, and let rest while you make the dressing.

3. In a small bowl, mix the remaining 3 tablespoons of lime juice, shallot, olive oil, and garlic. Season with salt.

4. Thinly slice the beef against the grain.

5. Toss the greens with the dressing and arrange on four plates. Garnish with the scallions and top with the sliced beef.

VARIATION TIP: Add any fresh herbs you like to expand on the flavors of the salad. Fresh thyme, cilantro, parsley, rosemary, and chives are all great herb additions in a green salad.

Per serving: Calories 358; Total fat 24g; Saturated fat 9g; Cholesterol 85mg; Carbs 9g; Fiber 3g; Protein 28g; Sodium 134mg

BEEF AND CHICKEN LIVER BURGERS

FLARE SOOTHER | FATIGUE-FRIENDLY | BONE BOOSTER

The difficult thing for many people when eating liver is its texture. It can be less than pleasant when prepared on its own, because cooked liver is often dry. But when you mix it with ground beef, you barely even know it's there, and it gives you a great boost of iron, B vitamins, and vitamin A.

SERVES 4

Prep time: 10 minutes

Cook time: 10 minutes

¼ pound chicken livers

½ cup roughly chopped red onion

1 pound ground beef

1 teaspoon sea salt

4 large lettuce leaves

1 cucumber, sliced

1. In a food processor, purée the livers and onion until smooth. Add the ground beef and salt, and pulse until it is all mixed well. Use your hands to form the meat into four burgers.

2. Heat a large skillet over medium heat and cook the burgers for 4 to 5 minutes on each side, flipping once, until cooked through.

3. Serve each burger on a lettuce leaf topped with cucumber slices.

VARIATION TIP: For something different, try stuffing the burgers with Nut-Free Basil Pesto (page 164). Form a burger and create an indentation in the center. Spoon in about 1 tablespoon of pesto, and fold and stretch the meat over to enclose the pesto. Cook as directed.

Per serving: Calories 229; Total fat 10g; Saturated fat 4g; Cholesterol 230mg; Carbs 5g; Fiber 1g; Protein 30g; Sodium 578mg

MARINATED BEEF HEART KEBABS

FATIGUE-FRIENDLY | CARDIO CARE | BONE BOOSTER

Working with beef heart is quite similar to most other cuts of meat. Be sure to cut it thin, as it soaks up the marinade better and helps create tender, delicious morsels of goodness. Serve the skewers with roasted vegetables (you can put them on skewers, too) or your favorite salad.

SERVES 6

Prep time: 10 minutes, plus at least 1 hour to marinate

Cook time: 10 minutes

1 (2- to 2½-pound) beef heart

3 garlic cloves, minced

2 tablespoons extra-virgin olive oil

Juice of 1 lemon or lime

1 fresh rosemary sprig, leaves removed and chopped

1 fresh thyme sprig, leaves removed and chopped

½ teaspoon sea salt

1. Trim away the tough fibers from around the heart and separate the flesh into ⅛-inch-thick, 2-inch-long pieces.

2. In a zip-top bag, combine the garlic, olive oil, lemon juice, rosemary, thyme, and salt. Add the meat and turn the pieces to coat them. Refrigerate for at least 1 hour or as long as overnight.

3. Preheat a grill to medium-high heat. Skewer the pieces onto metal skewers. Grill for 8 to 10 minutes, flipping once about halfway through, until browned but still medium inside. Or place a rack inside a rimmed baking sheet and broil in your oven for 8 to 10 minutes, flipping once about halfway through.

INGREDIENT TIP: Beef hearts are available at specialty grocery stores, Asian and Latin American markets, and directly from the butcher.

Per serving: Calories 292; Total fat 12g; Saturated fat 3g; Cholesterol 321mg; Carbs 1g; Fiber 0g; Protein 43g; Sodium 245mg

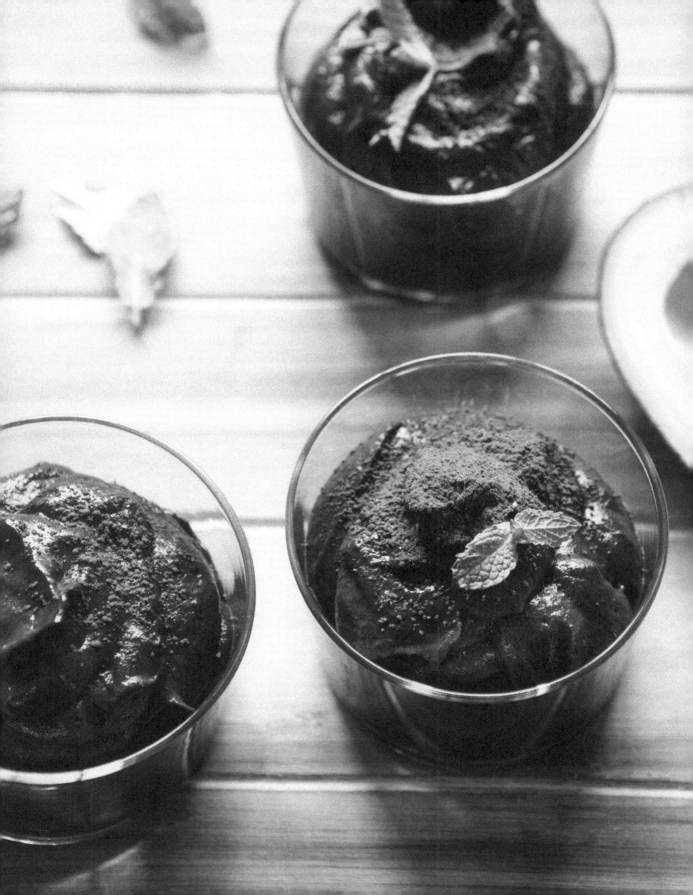

8

Desserts

BLACKBERRY MINT POPSICLES

FLARE SOOTHER	FATIGUE-FRIENDLY	KIDNEY SUPPORT	CARDIO CARE	BONE BOOSTER

There is not much that's easier to make for dessert than fresh frozen fruit pops that highlight the natural flavors of the season. If you have fresh blackberries, use them; if not, frozen work just as well. This fragrant summer combination captures the season on a stick.

MAKES 6

Prep time: 20 minutes, plus 3 to 4 hours to freeze

Cook time: 5 minutes

½ cup water

½ cup chopped mint leaves

2 tablespoons honey

2 cups blackberries

Juice of 1 lemon

1. In a small pot, bring the water to a boil over medium-high heat. Turn off the heat and add the mint leaves. Steep for 15 minutes. Add the honey and mix well to combine. Strain the leaves from the liquid and discard them.

2. In a blender, process the blackberries until smooth. Pour in the mint-honey water and the lemon juice. Mix to combine.

3. Pour into six popsicle molds. Insert the popsicle sticks into the molds and freeze for 3 to 4 hours until frozen through.

SUBSTITUTION TIP: Don't have honey? Try pure maple syrup instead. You can also substitute any other type of berry such as blueberries, strawberries, or raspberries.

Per serving: Calories 47; Total fat 0g; Saturated fat 0g; Cholesterol 0mg; Carbs 11g; Fiber 3g; Protein 1g; Sodium 6mg

PINEAPPLE COCONUT CREAMSICLES

FATIGUE-FRIENDLY | KIDNEY SUPPORT

It's fun to make these layered popsicles, giving you a break from the ordinary. If you have the time (and patience), you can freeze each layer for about 30 minutes before adding the next, to have well-defined layers—or you can carefully pour the different layers in without stirring for more loosely defined layers. Either way, these are fun tropical popsicles that are like a day at the beach.

MAKES 6

Prep time: 5 minutes,
plus 3 to 4 hours to freeze

2 cups chopped pineapple

1 cup coconut cream

1 teaspoon pure
vanilla extract

2 tablespoons honey

1. In a blender, process the pineapple until smooth.

2. In a small bowl, mix the coconut cream, vanilla extract, and honey.

3. Fill each of six popsicle molds ⅓ full with pineapple purée. Carefully pour the coconut cream mixture into the molds on top of the pineapple. Top each with the remaining pineapple. Insert the popsicle sticks into the molds and freeze for 3 to 4 hours until frozen through.

SUBSTITUTION TIP: Other tropical fruits, such as mango and papaya, taste great in place of the pineapple.

Per serving: Calories 193; Total fat 7g; Saturated fat 6g; Cholesterol 0mg; Carbs 34g; Fiber 1g; Protein 1g; Sodium 15mg

STRAWBERRY GRANITA

FLARE SOOTHER | FATIGUE-FRIENDLY | KIDNEY SUPPORT

A fruit granita is super easy to pull off and is so fun to eat. Kind of like a natural slushy, a granita is a great way to add fruit to your diet and keep you cool. Strawberries are loaded with vitamin C and provide great kidney support. Look for local strawberries in season for the best flavor, and try to buy organic to avoid pesticide exposure.

SERVES 6

Prep time: 5 minutes, plus 2½ hours to freeze

¼ cup honey

1 tablespoon freshly squeezed lemon juice

¾ cup hot water

1 pound strawberries, hulled

1. In a small bowl, mix the honey, lemon juice, and hot water. Stir until the honey is mixed.

2. In a blender, process the strawberries until smooth. Mix together with the honey syrup.

3. Transfer to a baking dish and freeze for 30 minutes. Using a fork, break the granita up and place back in the freezer. Continue to freeze for about 2 hours, breaking up with a fork every 30 minutes or so, until it has the texture of icy granules. Serve right away or cover tightly and freeze.

SUBSTITUTION TIP: Watermelon, cantaloupe, and pineapple all work great for a granita, as well.

Per serving: Calories 68; Total fat 0g; Saturated fat 0g; Cholesterol 0mg; Carbs 18g; Fiber 2g; Protein 1g; Sodium 2mg

CAROB FREEZER FUDGE

FLARE SOOTHER | FATIGUE-FRIENDLY | BONE BOOSTER

Freezer fudge is fun because you get all the luxuriousness of fudge with very little of the work. This is a quick mix-and-go recipe that only requires a bit of patience while the fudge sets in the freezer. The healthy fats in the coconut butter, coconut cream, and oil used here help nourish your body. This delicious treat is naturally sweet.

MAKES 16 SERVINGS (1 TABLESPOON EACH)

Prep time: 5 minutes, plus 1 to 2 hours to freeze

Cook time: 5 minutes

½ cup Coconut Butter (page 153)

¼ cup coconut cream

2 tablespoons coconut oil

2 tablespoons honey

2 tablespoons carob powder

1. In a small saucepan over medium heat, combine the coconut butter, coconut cream, coconut oil, honey, and carob powder. Stir to combine. When all the ingredients are mixed and melted, pour into a small pan or ice cube trays in 1-tablespoon portions.

2. Freeze until firm. Store for up to 7 days refrigerated in an airtight container, or freeze for up to 1 month.

STORAGE TIP: Be sure to always store this in the refrigerator or freezer. When left at room temperature it can melt. Eat the small pieces straight out of the freezer, or let them thaw for 5 to 10 minutes before eating.

Per serving: Calories 139; Total fat 12g; Saturated fat 10g; Cholesterol 0mg; Carbs 10g; Fiber 3g; Protein 1g; Sodium 7mg

MINT CHOCOLATE BOMBS

FLARE SOOTHER | FATIGUE-FRIENDLY | CARDIO CARE | BONE BOOSTER

This peppermint version of freezer fudge is simple and sweet. Because the base of the bombs is coconut oil, these treats will melt at room temperature during the hotter months, so be sure to store them in the refrigerator.

**MAKES 16 SERVINGS
(1 TABLESPOON EACH)**

Prep time: 5 minutes,
plus 1 to 2 hours to freeze

1 cup coconut oil

1 cup unsweetened dark cocoa powder

2 tablespoons pure maple syrup

Pinch sea salt

1 teaspoon peppermint extract

1. In a blender or food processor, combine the coconut oil, cocoa powder, maple syrup, salt, and peppermint extract. Blend well until smooth.

2. Transfer to ice cube trays or molds and freeze in 1-tablespoon portions. Once frozen, pop the pieces out and store them in the refrigerator or freezer in a zip-top bag or jar.

INGREDIENT TIP: Although chocolate, with its sugar and fat, is excluded from this diet, a small amount of plain cocoa powder is fine. Look for a peppermint extract that does not contain any fillers such as unhealthy oils or glycerin.

Per serving: Calories 137; Total fat 14g; Saturated fat 12g; Cholesterol 0mg; Carbs 5g; Fiber 2g; Protein 1g; Sodium 13mg

NO-BAKE CAROB BALLS

FATIGUE-FRIENDLY | BONE BOOSTER

These are great treats year round as they require no cooking, making them a perfect on-the-go sweet. Because they are loaded with healthy fats, they make as good an afternoon snack as they do a dessert.

MAKES 8

Prep time: 5 minutes, plus 1 hour to chill

1 cup Coconut Butter (page 153)

½ cup unsweetened shredded coconut, plus more for rolling

1 tablespoon coconut oil

1 tablespoon carob powder

1. Soften the coconut butter, if necessary, to stir. In a medium mixing bowl, combine the coconut butter, shredded coconut, coconut oil, and carob powder, and mix well.

2. Form into eight balls about 1 inch in diameter and roll the balls in additional coconut. Place them on a baking sheet or plate and refrigerate for 1 hour until firm.

3. Serve, or store in an airtight container refrigerated for up to 5 days.

INGREDIENT TIP: Carob powder is ground from carob pods, which are commonly used as a chocolate substitute. Unlike chocolate, carob doesn't contain caffeine or oxalic acid, and it is naturally sweet. Look for it in health food stores in the baking section.

Per serving: Calories 214; Total fat 21g; Saturated fat 20g; Cholesterol 0mg; Carbs 10g; Fiber 3g; Protein 3g; Sodium 6mg

COCONUT DATE BITES

FATIGUE-FRIENDLY | BONE BOOSTER

No-bake desserts are great because so little work is involved. Here, dates bring a lot of natural sweetness and work as a simple binder. Dates are a great source of B vitamins, iron, potassium, and magnesium, making them a healthy addition to your dessert lineup.

MAKES 12

Prep time: 10 minutes, plus 1 hour to chill

1 cup pitted dates

⅓ cup coconut oil

½ cup unsweetened shredded coconut, plus more for rolling

½ teaspoon sea salt

1 teaspoon ground cinnamon

1. In a food processor, combine the dates, coconut oil, coconut, salt, and cinnamon. Process until the mixture is uniformly ground and mixed.

2. Using your hands, shape the mixture into 12 small balls, about 1 inch in diameter. Roll the balls in additional coconut and place the balls on a baking sheet or plate and refrigerate for 1 hour until firm.

3. Serve, or store in an airtight container refrigerated for up to 5 days.

COOKING TIP: When you form the balls, depending on the room temperature where you are working, they may hold together firmly or loosely. Once the balls go in the refrigerator, the coconut oil will solidify and hold them together.

Per serving: Calories 122; Total fat 9g; Saturated fat 8g; Cholesterol 0mg; Carbs 12g; Fiber 2g; Protein 1g; Sodium 80mg

CREAMY CHOCOLATE AVOCADO PUDDING

FLARE SOOTHER | **FATIGUE-FRIENDLY** | **CARDIO CARE** | **BONE BOOSTER**

If you think an avocado makes a smoothie taste luxurious, you will love what it does to pudding. This healthy version of classic chocolate pudding is loaded with heart-healthy fats and tastes amazing.

SERVES 4

Prep time: 5 minutes

2 ripe avocados, pitted and peeled

¼ cup coconut milk

¼ cup unsweetened dark cocoa powder

2 tablespoons honey

1 teaspoon vanilla extract

Pinch sea salt

1. In a food processor, purée the avocados until smooth.

2. Add the coconut milk, cocoa powder, honey, vanilla, and salt. Process until smooth, about 2 minutes, and serve.

INGREDIENT TIP: Use the widely available Hass variety of avocado for making pudding. These are the creamiest and the best choice for this recipe. Look for avocados that yield to pressure when you gently squeeze them but are not overly soft.

Per serving: Calories 226; Total fat 18g; Saturated fat 5g; Cholesterol 0mg; Carbs 20g; Fiber 8g; Protein 3g; Sodium 69mg

RASPBERRY MOUSSE

| FLARE SOOTHER | FATIGUE-FRIENDLY | KIDNEY SUPPORT | CARDIO CARE |

Raspberries create a beautifully colored and delicately flavored mousse, and coconut cream is the perfect whipped substitute for cream. Raspberries are rich in antioxidants and support the kidneys, making them a great sweet treat. After a long day, this is one perfectly healthy way to unwind and treat yourself.

SERVES 4

Prep time: 10 minutes

1 cup raspberries, plus more for serving

1 (14-ounce) can coconut milk, chilled

2 tablespoons pure maple syrup

1 teaspoon freshly squeezed lime juice

1. In a blender, purée the raspberries until smooth.

2. Open the can of coconut milk without shaking. Scrape the coconut cream from the top into a mixing bowl, leaving the watery part behind. Beat the coconut cream by hand or using an electric mixer for 2 minutes until thickened.

3. Add the maple syrup and continue to mix. Add the lime juice. Beat on low for 1 minute. Fold in the raspberries until just mixed. Serve immediately.

SUBSTITUTION TIP: Strawberries and blackberries will also work well in this recipe.

Per serving: Calories 273; Total fat 24g; Saturated fat 21g; Cholesterol 0mg; Carbs 17g; Fiber 4g; Protein 3g; Sodium 16mg

PUMPKIN PARFAIT

FLARE SOOTHER | FATIGUE-FRIENDLY | CARDIO CARE

If you want to capture fall in a glass, this is the dessert for you. If you are not eating this right away, hold off on adding the coconut chips until just before serving. That way, the chips will stay crisp and create a nice contrast in textures.

SERVES 4

Prep time: 10 minutes

2 cups plain pumpkin purée

1 teaspoon ground cinnamon

1 teaspoon ground ginger

2 tablespoons pure maple syrup

¼ teaspoon sea salt

1 (14-ounce) can full-fat coconut milk, chilled

½ cup toasted coconut chips

1. In a blender, process the pumpkin purée, cinnamon, ginger, maple syrup, and salt until smooth.

2. Open the can of coconut milk without shaking. Scrape the coconut cream from the top into a mixing bowl, leaving the watery part behind. Beat the coconut cream by hand or using an electric mixer for 2 minutes until thickened.

3. Spoon about ¼ cup of pumpkin mixture into four glasses. Top each with a spoonful of coconut cream. Divide the remaining pumpkin purée into the glasses, and top with the remaining coconut cream. Top each parfait with 2 tablespoons of toasted coconut and serve.

INGREDIENT TIP: To toast coconut chips, spread them in a thin layer and place in the oven at 325°F for 5 to 10 minutes, stirring once or twice, until brown and toasted. They will toast quickly, so don't wander away from the kitchen while they cook.

Per serving: Calories 348; Total fat 29g; Saturated fat 25g; Cholesterol 0mg; Carbs 25g; Fiber 7g; Protein 4g; Sodium 142mg

BUTTERNUT SPICE COOKIES

FLARE SOOTHER | FATIGUE-FRIENDLY | CARDIO CARE

Even butternut squash can become dessert in these tasty spiced cookies. Cinnamon and ginger give the cookies a ginger-snap feel, while the squash gives you plenty of veggie fiber and vitamins to make this a cookie you can feel good about eating.

MAKES ABOUT 12 COOKIES

Prep time: 10 minutes

Cook time: 10 minutes

1 cup cooked mashed butternut squash

¼ cup honey

1 tablespoon Coconut Butter (page 153)

2 tablespoons coconut oil

2 tablespoons coconut flour

½ cup arrowroot powder

1 teaspoon ground cinnamon

½ teaspoon baking soda

¼ teaspoon ground ginger

¼ teaspoon sea salt

1. Preheat the oven to 375°F. Line a baking sheet with parchment paper.

2. In a large mixing bowl, combine the squash, honey, coconut butter, and coconut oil. Mix well.

3. Stir in the coconut flour, arrowroot powder, cinnamon, baking soda, ginger, and salt. Mix well.

4. Scoop up tablespoon-size pieces of the dough and place on a baking sheet, leaving about 2 inches of space between each cookie.

5. Bake for 8 to 10 minutes until just lightly browned.

SUBSTITUTION TIP: You can substitute plain pumpkin purée for the butternut squash.

Per serving: Calories 97; Total fat 4g; Saturated fat 4g; Cholesterol 0mg; Carbs 15g; Fiber 2g; Protein 1g; Sodium 93mg

OVEN-POACHED PEARS

FLARE SOOTHER | FATIGUE-FRIENDLY | KIDNEY SUPPORT

When you cut out processed sugars, it can be amazing how wonderfully sweet natural sugars taste. Pears are elevated to dessert status with just a few tweaks and a little basting in this simple, cinnamon-kissed fruit dessert.

SERVES 4

Prep time: 5 minutes
Cook time: 45 minutes

2 firm pears

2 tablespoons freshly squeezed lemon juice

1 tablespoon honey

1 tablespoon coconut oil

1-inch piece fresh ginger, sliced

½ cup water

1 cinnamon stick

1. Preheat the oven to 400°F.

2. Peel the pears and use a spoon to scrape out the core from the bottom, removing the seeds. Stand the pears upright in a baking dish, cutting a piece from the bottom of the pears, if necessary.

3. In a medium bowl, mix the lemon juice, honey, coconut oil, and ginger. Add the water and mix well to dissolve the honey.

4. Pour the liquid over the pears and add the cinnamon stick. Cover the baking dish with aluminum foil and bake for 45 minutes total. After 15 minutes, baste some of the liquid over the pears, and continue to do so every 10 to 15 minutes during cooking.

5. Serve immediately or refrigerate along with the liquid and serve cold.

INGREDIENT TIP: Anjou, Bartlett, and Bosc are all great varieties for poaching as they hold up well to long cooking.

Per serving: Calories 108; Total fat 4g; Saturated fat 3g; Cholesterol 0mg; Carbs 20g; Fiber 3g; Protein 1g; Sodium 3mg

LEMON TART

FLARE SOOTHER | FATIGUE-FRIENDLY | BONE BOOSTER

If you like the tang of a lemon tart, this version will not disappoint. Using naturally sweet coconut and sweet and sticky dates, the crust is super easy, no-bake, and gluten-free. The lemon custard is rich with coconut milk and just lightly sweetened with honey, for a wonderful tart-sweet combination.

SERVES 8

Prep time: 10 minutes, plus 2½ hours to chill

Cook time: 10 minutes

1½ cups unsweetened shredded coconut

1 cup pitted dates, coarsely chopped

3 tablespoons unflavored gelatin

½ cup water

Zest and juice of 4 lemons

1 (14-ounce) can coconut milk

¼ cup honey

1. Preheat the oven to 350°F.

2. In a food processor, combine the coconut and dates and pulse several times until the dates are well chopped. Transfer the mixture to the bottom of a 9-inch pie dish or a springform pan and use your hands to press it evenly into the dish. Refrigerate until firm, about 10 minutes. Transfer to the oven and bake for 10 minutes until browned. Let cool completely.

3. While the crust is baking, in a small saucepan, combine the gelatin and water and stir until the gelatin is completely dissolved. Let sit for about 3 minutes. Add the lemon juice and zest, coconut milk, and honey, and heat over medium heat until the honey and gelatin are completely dissolved. Turn off the heat.

4. Let everything rest for about 20 minutes while the crust cools, until the gelatin mixture is cool to the touch and beginning to thicken. Pour over the crust and carefully transfer to the refrigerator. Chill for at least 2 hours before serving.

VARIATION TIP: This tart can also be made using lime juice and zest. Use six limes in place of the four lemons.

Per serving: Calories 241; Total fat 14g; Saturated fat 12g; Cholesterol 0mg; Carbs 29g; Fiber 3g; Protein 4g; Sodium 19mg

BERRY COBBLER

| FLARE SOOTHER | FATIGUE-FRIENDLY | KIDNEY SUPPORT | CARDIO CARE | BONE BOOSTER |

Berry cobbler is an easy dessert that just oozes with wonderfulness every time you make it. Berries are an antioxidant powerhouse and perfect for including in your desserts. Because the natural sweetness becomes concentrated as the berries cook, the only sweetener used here is in the coconut flour topping.

SERVES 8

Prep time: 10 minutes

Cook time: 40 minutes

2 tablespoons coconut oil, softened, plus more for greasing

4 cups fresh or frozen berries (blackberries, blueberries, raspberries)

½ cup coconut flour

¼ cup honey

¼ teaspoon sea salt

½ teaspoon baking soda

1 tablespoon freshly squeezed lemon juice

2 tablespoons water

1. Preheat the oven to 300°F. Grease an 8-inch baking dish with a little coconut oil.

2. Spread the berries evenly in the bottom of the dish.

3. In a medium mixing bowl, combine the coconut oil, coconut flour, honey, salt, baking soda, lemon juice, and water. Mix by hand or using an electric mixer on medium. Spread the mixture in clumps over the berries.

4. Bake for 35 to 40 minutes until the top is golden brown.

SUBSTITUTION TIP: Use any fresh berries or fruit in season, or use frozen instead. Nectarines, peaches, strawberries, rhubarb, and apples all work well in this simple cobbler.

Per serving: Calories 154; Total fat 5g; Saturated fat 4g; Cholesterol 0mg; Carbs 26g; Fiber 10g; Protein 3g; Sodium 139mg

SKILLET PEACH CRUMBLE

FLARE SOOTHER | FATIGUE-FRIENDLY | KIDNEY SUPPORT

This warming dessert uses arrowroot powder for the crumble—another great alternative to grain toppings. Peaches are cleansing to the kidneys and are a good source of vitamins A and C. Cinnamon and maple syrup give the peaches even more great flavor in this simple yet delicious dessert.

SERVES 8

Prep time: 10 minutes

Cook time: 30 minutes

4 cups fresh or frozen peach slices, thawed

¼ cup pure maple syrup

1 teaspoon freshly squeezed lemon juice

¼ teaspoon ground cinnamon

2 teaspoons arrowroot powder, plus 1 cup

½ teaspoon sea salt

½ teaspoon baking soda

¼ cup coconut oil, melted

1. Preheat the oven to 425°F.

2. In a large mixing bowl, combine the peaches, maple syrup, lemon juice, cinnamon, and 2 teaspoons of the arrowroot powder. Pour the mixture into a medium oven-safe skillet. Bake for 10 minutes.

3. While the peaches are cooking, in a medium mixing bowl, combine the remaining 1 cup of arrowroot powder, salt, baking soda, and coconut oil. Mix well and add 2 to 3 tablespoons of water to the mixture until the dough comes together.

4. Crumble the dough over the top of the peaches in the skillet to cover them. Bake for an additional 15 to 20 minutes until browned.

SUBSTITUTION TIP: Use this recipe with any other stone fruits, such as nectarines or plums.

Per serving: Calories 180; Total fat 7g; Saturated fat 6g; Cholesterol 0mg; Carbs 29g; Fiber 1g; Protein 1g; Sodium 197mg

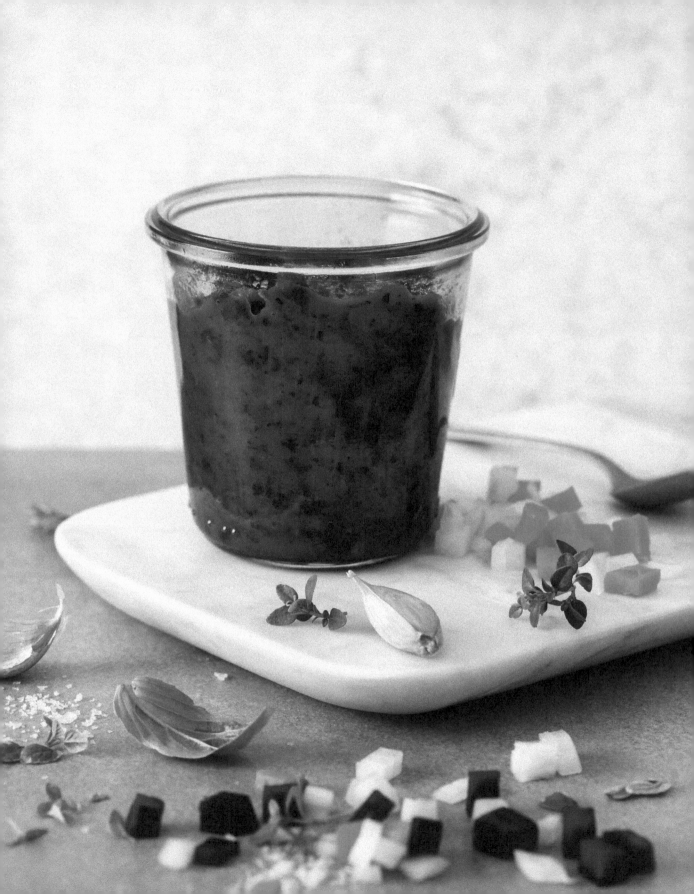

9

Broths, Basics, Dressings, and Sauces

VEGETABLE BROTH

| FLARE SOOTHER | FATIGUE-FRIENDLY | KIDNEY SUPPORT | CARDIO CARE | BONE BOOSTER |

This simple vegetable broth has tons of flavor yet is neutral enough to complement the taste of whatever you cook with it. You will love adding it to your favorite dishes to boost the flavor and the nutrients. To save on vegetables, keep the scraps you trim (the ends of onions, carrots, celery) in the freezer until you have enough saved to make this broth.

MAKES ABOUT 8 CUPS

Prep time: 5 minutes

Cook time: 1 hour

1 large onion

2 large carrots

3 celery stalks

1 bunch fresh parsley

1 bay leaf

1. Chop all the vegetables into medium chunks and place in a large pot.

2. Cover the vegetables with a couple of inches of water and bring to a simmer over medium-high heat. Reduce the heat to medium-low.

3. Cook for about 1 hour, uncovered, until the stock is reduced slightly and just golden. Strain and discard the vegetables.

4. Transfer to smaller containers, cool, and store in the refrigerator for up to 5 days, or for up to 3 months in the freezer.

VARIATION TIP: You can also freeze any broth in ice-cube trays, and store the frozen cubes in a zip-top freezer bag. This way, you will always have small amounts of broth on hand for quick additions to sauces and stews.

Per serving (1 cup): Calories 10; Total fat 0g; Saturated fat 0g; Cholesterol 0mg; Carbs 3g; Fiber 0g; Protein 0g; Sodium 20mg

CHICKEN BONE BROTH

| FLARE SOOTHER | FATIGUE-FRIENDLY | KIDNEY SUPPORT | CARDIO CARE | BONE BOOSTER |

Bone broth is the cornerstone of so many recipes in this book. It is one of the best homemade remedies around for healing the gut, and if you follow the recipes in this book, you are going to want to make this broth yourself. You can buy bone broth in a health food store, but this flavorful version is so easy to make at home and is more nutritious than most store-bought versions. You can use the picked-over carcass from a store-bought rotisserie chicken as the base. Add a sprig of your favorite herbs to give the broth even more flavor. Thyme, oregano, parsley, and tarragon all add a level of complexity to this broth.

MAKES ABOUT 8 CUPS

Prep time: 5 minutes

Cook time: 5 hours

1 whole chicken carcass (just the bones)

2 celery stalks, chopped into a few pieces

2 carrots, chopped into a few pieces

1 onion, halved

1 tablespoon apple cider vinegar

1 fresh herb sprig (thyme, oregano, parsley, tarragon)

1. In a large stockpot, combine the chicken carcass, celery, carrots, onion, vinegar, and herb. Cover with water so the chicken carcass and vegetables are covered by a few inches of water.

2. Bring to a boil, reduce the heat to the lowest setting, partially cover, and simmer for at least 5 hours. If the broth reduces below the level of the bones and vegetables, add a bit more water to the pot so they remain covered.

3. Strain the solids and discard.

4. Transfer to smaller containers, cool, and store in the refrigerator for up to 4 days, or for up to 2 months in the freezer.

COOKING TIP: If you don't want to leave your stock simmering on the stove all day, make it in a slow cooker instead. Follow the same instructions and cook it for 8 to 12 hours on low.

Per serving (1 cup): Calories 35; Total fat 1g; Saturated fat 0g; Cholesterol 0mg; Carbs 3g; Fiber 0g; Protein 2g; Sodium 87mg

BEEF BONE BROTH

| FLARE SOOTHER | FATIGUE-FRIENDLY | KIDNEY SUPPORT | CARDIO CARE | BONE BOOSTER |

Beef bone broth really benefits from a longer cook time than chicken, so for this recipe, we recommend using a slow cooker to make it an easy hands-off experience. For added flavor and richness in the finished broth, we roast the bones first. You can skip this step, but be sure to still rinse the bones first before using. Look for beef marrow bones in the frozen or fresh meat section of your grocery store, or get them directly from a butcher.

MAKES ABOUT 8 CUPS

Prep time: 5 minutes

Cook time: 12 to 24 hours

2 pounds beef marrow bones

1 tablespoon apple cider vinegar

1 carrot, chopped into a few pieces

1 large onion, halved

1. Preheat the oven to 400°F.

2. Rinse the bones under cold water and arrange in a single layer on a rimmed baking sheet. Roast for about 30 minutes until browned.

3. Transfer the bones to a slow cooker and add the vinegar, carrot, and onion. Cover with water by a few inches. Cook on high for 12 to 24 hours.

4. Strain the broth, discarding the bones.

5. Transfer to smaller containers, cool, and store in the refrigerator for up to 5 days, or for up to 3 months in the freezer.

COOKING TIP: Rinsing the bones under cool water removes blood from them, resulting in a clearer broth.

Per serving: Calories 20; Total fat 1g; Saturated fat 0g; Cholesterol 0mg; Carbs 1g; Fiber 0g; Protein 2g; Sodium 78mg

COCONUT BUTTER

FATIGUE-FRIENDLY | KIDNEY SUPPORT

Coconut butter is a thick and luscious condiment that contains both coconut shreds and oil to create a spreadable end result. You can use it in baking or spread it on a warm sweet potato, green beans, or corn. It is versatile, delicious, and so good you could almost eat it on its own.

MAKES ABOUT 2 CUPS (2 TABLESPOONS PER SERVING)

Prep time: 10 minutes

2 cups unsweetened shredded coconut

4 tablespoons coconut oil, divided

1. In a high-speed blender or food processor, combine the coconut and 2 tablespoons of the coconut oil. Process on high for 3 to 10 minutes until smooth, scraping down the sides a couple of times throughout. If needed, add the additional 2 tablespoons of coconut oil to create a smooth butter.

2. Store in an airtight container at room temperature.

VARIATION TIP: If desired, add up to 1 tablespoon of honey or pure maple syrup for some sweetness.

Per serving: Calories 111; Total fat 11g; Saturated fat 11g; Cholesterol 0mg; Carbs 6g; Fiber 1g; Protein 2g; Sodium 0mg

CREAMY EGG-FREE MAYO

Use this to make the Chicken Salad with Apple and Grapes (page 116), or just for dipping vegetables—it is really that tasty all on its own. After sitting, the oils will separate; simply stir before using to combine them again.

MAKES ABOUT ½ CUP (2 TABLESPOONS PER SERVING)

Prep time: 5 minutes

¼ cup Coconut Butter (page 153)

4 tablespoons extra-virgin olive oil

½ teaspoon garlic powder

1 teaspoon apple cider vinegar

1 teaspoon freshly squeezed lemon juice

¼ teaspoon sea salt

2 tablespoons warm water

1. In a blender or food processor, combine all the ingredients, and process until smooth.

2. Transfer to an airtight jar and store in the refrigerator for up to 5 days.

VARIATION TIP: Add fresh herbs such as cilantro, parsley, mint, or oregano to suit your tastes. Simply chop the herbs finely and stir them into the finished mayo.

Per serving: Calories 178; Total fat 20g; Saturated fat 8g; Cholesterol 0mg; Carbs 3g; Fiber 0g; Protein 1g; Sodium 117mg

BALSAMIC VINAIGRETTE

FLARE SOOTHER | FATIGUE-FRIENDLY | KIDNEY SUPPORT | CARDIO CARE

It's always helpful to have a go-to dressing on hand for quick salads throughout the week. This simple vinaigrette comes together in just minutes and works on a green salad and as a marinade. Keep it in a jar in plain sight in your kitchen and you will find yourself eating more salads; it is fine to store at room temperature.

MAKES ABOUT ¾ CUP (2 TABLESPOONS PER SERVING)

Prep time: 5 minutes

½ cup extra-virgin olive oil

3 tablespoons balsamic vinegar

1 teaspoon honey

Sea salt

Freshly ground black pepper

1. In a small jar, whisk together the olive oil, vinegar, and honey. Season with salt and pepper.

2. Screw the lid on the jar and store at room temperature.

VARIATION TIP: Add any combination of fresh ingredients to the vinaigrette, such as herbs, garlic, shallots, or scallions. Be sure to refrigerate the finished vinaigrette if fresh ingredients are included.

Per serving: Calories 149; Total fat 17g; Saturated fat 2g; Cholesterol 0mg; Carbs 1g; Fiber 0g; Protein 0g; Sodium 39mg

GARLIC-CILANTRO VINAIGRETTE

FLARE SOOTHER | **FATIGUE-FRIENDLY** | **KIDNEY SUPPORT** | **CARDIO CARE**

This bright vinaigrette is like summer in a jar. Cilantro is a great digestive aid, and the bonus is that it brightens so many dishes so well. Use this on a fresh green salad or to marinate vegetables or meat before grilling or roasting.

MAKES ABOUT ½ CUP (2 TABLESPOONS PER SERVING)

Prep time: 5 minutes

¼ cup extra-virgin olive oil

2 tablespoons apple cider vinegar

½ cup chopped fresh cilantro leaves and stems

2 garlic cloves, peeled

1 teaspoon honey

½ teaspoon onion powder

2 tablespoons water

Sea salt

1. In a blender, combine the olive oil, vinegar, cilantro, garlic, honey, onion powder, and water. Process until smooth. Season with salt.

2. Store in an airtight container for up to 3 days in the refrigerator.

SUBSTITUTION TIP: You can substitute parsley for the cilantro.

Per serving: Calories 118; Total fat 13g; Saturated fat 2g; Cholesterol 0mg; Carbs 2g; Fiber 0g; Protein 0g; Sodium 59mg

CREAMY CAESAR DRESSING

| FLARE SOOTHER | FATIGUE-FRIENDLY | KIDNEY SUPPORT | CARDIO CARE | BONE BOOSTER |

It can be really hard to give up simple conveniences such as bottled dressings and dips. With this easy and quick dressing, you won't feel like you are missing out at all. If the idea of anchovy paste makes you squeamish, please do try it in this dressing. It gives Caesar dressing its characteristic flavor and really doesn't make it taste fishy at all.

MAKES ABOUT ¾ CUP (2 TABLESPOONS PER SERVING)

Prep time: 5 minutes

½ cup avocado oil

2 tablespoons extra-virgin olive oil

Juice of 1 lemon

1 teaspoon fish sauce

3 garlic cloves, peeled

1 teaspoon anchovy paste

¼ teaspoon sea salt

1. In a blender, combine all the ingredients, and process until smooth.

2. Use immediately or transfer to an airtight storage container and refrigerate for up to 3 days.

VARIATION TIP: This is also really good with fresh herbs added. Depending on what you are serving it with, either cilantro or basil can turn this into a wonderfully flavorful herby dressing.

Per serving: Calories 207; Total fat 24g; Saturated fat 4g; Cholesterol 3mg; Carbs 1g; Fiber 0g; Protein 0g; Sodium 209mg

OLIVE TAPENADE

FLARE SOOTHER | FATIGUE-FRIENDLY | KIDNEY SUPPORT

A flavorful mix of olives and capers, this lovely tapenade can be stirred into a salad or used as a dip for vegetables. With the fresh combination of parsley, basil, and oregano, the tapenade is bright and fragrant.

MAKES ABOUT 1 CUP (2 TABLESPOONS PER SERVING)

Prep time: 5 minutes

2 cups pitted brined black olives (such as Kalamata or Niçoise)

2 tablespoons capers, rinsed

2 garlic cloves, peeled

Juice of 1 lemon

2 tablespoons chopped fresh parsley leaves

1 tablespoon chopped fresh basil leaves

1 teaspoon chopped fresh oregano leaves

¼ cup extra-virgin olive oil

1. In a food processor, pulse the olives, capers, and garlic in 2-second intervals, until the olives are broken down into small pieces. Scrape down the sides of the bowl.

2. Add the lemon juice, parsley, basil, oregano, and olive oil. Pulse again until the herbs are just chopped, scraping down the sides of the bowl.

3. Store in an airtight container in the refrigerator for up to 1 week.

SUBSTITUTION TIP: If you don't have fresh parsley, basil, and oregano, use about 2 teaspoons of dried parsley and 1 teaspoon each of dried basil and oregano.

Per serving: Calories 114; Total fat 11g; Saturated fat 1g; Cholesterol 0mg, Carbs 3g; Fiber 0g; Protein 0g; Sodium 278mg

MANGO CHUTNEY

FLARE SOOTHER | FATIGUE-FRIENDLY | KIDNEY SUPPORT | CARDIO CARE

The combination of sweet and savory is a central feature of this simple chutney that skips the spice. This sticky, thick chutney makes a great topping for grilled fish and also goes well with pork and chicken. Make a jar to have on hand to dress up any meal.

MAKES ABOUT 1½ CUPS (2 TABLESPOONS PER SERVING)

Prep time: 10 minutes

Cook time: 7 minutes

1 tablespoon coconut oil

½ cup chopped red onion

1 tablespoon minced fresh garlic

1 tablespoon minced fresh ginger

2 mangos, peeled and chopped, or 2 cups frozen mango, thawed

Juice of 2 limes

2 tablespoons apple cider vinegar

Sea salt

1. In a large skillet, heat the coconut oil over medium heat. Cook the onion, garlic, and ginger for 2 minutes, stirring constantly.

2. Add the mango, lime juice, and vinegar, and cook for about 5 minutes until softened. Let cool and season with salt.

3. Store unused chutney in an airtight container in the refrigerator for up to 5 days.

VARIATION TIP: If you like raisins, add ¼ cup of golden raisins with the other ingredients in step 2 to increase the sweetness and give it another dimension.

Per serving: Calories 49; Total fat 1g; Saturated fat 1g; Cholesterol 0mg; Carbs 10g; Fiber 1g; Protein 1g; Sodium 21mg

PEACH SALSA

Peaches have just enough sweetness to make a wonderfully complex salsa. Like the Mango Chutney (page 159), this works well with fish, chicken, and pork. Be sure to use ripe peaches that are ready to eat.

**MAKES ABOUT 2 CUPS
(¼ CUP PER SERVING)**

Prep time: 10 minutes

3 ripe peaches, pitted
and diced

3 scallions, chopped

2 garlic cloves, minced

1 tablespoon freshly
squeezed lime juice

1 tablespoon extra-virgin
olive oil

½ cup chopped fresh
cilantro leaves

Sea salt

1. In a large bowl, mix the peaches, scallions, garlic, lime juice, olive oil, and cilantro. Season with salt.

2. Transfer to a jar and store in the refrigerator for up to 5 days.

SUBSTITUTION TIP: You can substitute about ¼ cup of chopped red onion for the scallions.

Per serving: Calories 42; Total fat 2g; Saturated fat 0g; Cholesterol 0mg; Carbs 6g; Fiber 1g; Protein 1g; Sodium 33mg

PUMPKIN DIP

FLARE SOOTHER | **FATIGUE-FRIENDLY**

Pumpkin purée is often found in sweet dishes, but with this recipe you will see how great it tastes savory. Anti-inflammatory turmeric blends right in along with the warming cinnamon for this wonderful dip loaded with vegetable power. Use it alongside fresh vegetables or for dunking Jicama Oven Fries (page 52).

SERVES 2

Prep time: 5 minutes

1 cup plain pumpkin purée

1 small zucchini or yellow summer squash

Juice of 1 lemon

2 tablespoons extra-virgin olive oil

2 garlic cloves, chopped

½-inch piece fresh ginger, peeled and roughly chopped

1 teaspoon ground cinnamon

1 teaspoon ground turmeric

1. In a blender or food processor, combine all the ingredients, and process until smooth.

2. Transfer to a jar and store in the refrigerator for up to 3 days.

INGREDIENT TIP: Be sure to purchase pumpkin purée and not pumpkin pie filling. The labels look similar, but the pie filling is loaded with spices and sugar.

Per serving: Calories 193; Total fat 15g; Saturated fat 3g; Cholesterol 0mg; Carbs 16g; Fiber 6g; Protein 3g; Sodium 18mg

CAULI-RANCH DIP

FLARE SOOTHER | FATIGUE-FRIENDLY | KIDNEY SUPPORT

Use this as a dip for raw veggie sticks such as cucumbers, celery, and carrots, or toss it with some crisp romaine for a tasty salad. Dress it up with even more herbs, if you like. A couple of sprigs of oregano, or cilantro or basil leaves, can easily give you a new take on this flavorful veggie-forward dip.

SERVES 2

Prep time: 5 minutes

2 cups frozen cauliflower florets, defrosted

1 cup coconut milk

½ teaspoon sea salt

½ teaspoon garlic powder

½ teaspoon onion powder

2 tablespoons chopped fresh parsley

2 fresh thyme sprigs, leaves removed and chopped

1. In a blender, combine all the ingredients, and process until smooth.

2. Transfer to a jar and store in the refrigerator for up to 3 days.

SUBSTITUTION TIP: If you don't have fresh herbs, use about 2 teaspoons of dried parsley and 1 teaspoon of dried thyme in place of the fresh.

Per serving: Calories 307; Total fat 29g; Saturated fat 25g; Cholesterol 0mg; Carbs 12g; Fiber 5g; Protein 5g; Sodium 509mg

CHIMICHURRI SAUCE

| FLARE SOOTHER | FATIGUE-FRIENDLY | KIDNEY SUPPORT | CARDIO CARE | BONE BOOSTER |

This Argentine sauce is perfect poured over meats, or you can drizzle it on cooked vegetables for a little extra nourishment and to brighten any meal. The traditional version contains red pepper for heat; it is omitted here, but the sauce is still loaded with flavor. The main component, parsley, is a digestive aid and helps support the kidneys, bladder, and stomach.

MAKES ABOUT ½ CUP (2 TABLESPOONS PER SERVING)

Prep time: 5 minutes

½ cup coarsely chopped fresh parsley

2 tablespoons chopped fresh oregano leaves

2 tablespoons apple cider vinegar

3 garlic cloves, minced

⅓ cup extra-virgin olive oil

Sea salt

1. In a blender, combine the parsley, oregano, vinegar, and garlic and process until smooth. (If needed, add a tablespoon or two of water or bone broth to create a smooth paste.)

2. Transfer to a bowl and pour the olive oil over the paste. Let rest for 30 minutes, stir well, and season with salt.

3. Transfer to a jar and store in the refrigerator for up to 3 days.

INGREDIENT TIP: There are two types of parsley commonly sold: curly and flatleaf (also known as Italian). Choose the Italian parsley for all the recipes in this book. This darker variety is much more flavorful and best for cooking, while the curly variety is great for garnish.

Per serving: Calories 154; Total fat 17g; Saturated fat 2g; Cholesterol 0mg; Carbs 2g; Fiber 0g; Protein 0g; Sodium 63mg

NUT-FREE BASIL PESTO

| FLARE SOOTHER | FATIGUE-FRIENDLY | KIDNEY SUPPORT | CARDIO CARE | BONE BOOSTER |

Most premade pestos contain a combination of nuts and cheese. Since both can be inflammatory, this alternative is a great way to still get all the wonderful flavors of this Italian condiment without sacrificing your health. Nutritional yeast, a deactivated yeast strain, provides a cheesy, nutty flavor that gives this sauce its characteristic appeal. It is available at specialty and health food stores.

MAKES ABOUT 1 CUP
(¼ CUP PER SERVING)

Prep time: 5 minutes

2 cups tightly packed fresh basil leaves

⅓ cup extra-virgin olive oil

Juice of 1 lemon

2 tablespoons nutritional yeast

2 garlic cloves, peeled

¼ teaspoon sea salt

1. In a blender, combine all the ingredients, and process until smooth. If necessary, add a couple of tablespoons of water or bone broth to create a smooth pesto.

2. Store in the refrigerator in an airtight container for up to 5 days.

SUBSTITUTION TIP: Another great base for pesto is arugula. Its bitter flavor is even tastier when accentuated with garlic and lemon. Use an equal amount of arugula in place of the basil for a zesty twist.

Per serving: Calories 182; Total fat 18g; Saturated fat 3g; Cholesterol 0mg; Carbs 5g; Fiber 2g; Protein 6g; Sodium 123mg

TOMATO-FREE MARINARA SAUCE

FLARE SOOTHER | FATIGUE-FRIENDLY | CARDIO CARE | BONE BOOSTER

If you miss your old favorite marinara sauce, try this substitute. Serve it over veggie noodles or along with Coconut Chicken Strips (page 117) as a dipping sauce.

MAKES 4 CUPS (1 CUP PER SERVING)

Prep time: 5 minutes

Cook time: 50 minutes

1 tablespoon extra-virgin olive oil

2 medium onions, chopped

3 garlic cloves, minced

1 pound carrots, chopped

1 large beet, peeled and chopped

1 cup Chicken Bone Broth (page 151)

1 fresh oregano sprig, leaves removed and chopped

1 fresh thyme sprig, leaves removed and chopped

½ teaspoon sea salt

Juice of 2 lemons

1 tablespoon chopped fresh basil

1. In a large pot, heat the olive oil over medium heat. Cook the onions for 5 to 7 minutes until softened and browned. Add the garlic and cook for 30 more seconds until fragrant.

2. Add the carrots, beet, broth, oregano, and thyme. Bring to a boil, lower the heat to medium-low, cover, and simmer for 30 to 40 minutes until the carrots and beet are fork tender.

3. Using an immersion blender or in a traditional blender, purée the sauce. Add the salt, lemon juice, and basil

COOKING TIP: Too much sauce? You can keep it in the refrigerator for about 5 days. If you are not going to eat it by then, freeze the extra for up to 2 months.

Per serving: Calories 118; Total fat 4g; Saturated fat 1g; Cholesterol 0mg; Carbs 20g; Fiber 5g; Protein 3g; Sodium 307mg

CHERRY BARBECUE SAUCE

FLARE SOOTHER | FATIGUE-FRIENDLY | KIDNEY SUPPORT | CARDIO CARE

Barbecue sauce is not off the menu when you have this delicious cherry-based version on hand. Loaded with vitamin C plus antioxidant and anti-inflammatory compounds, cherries are a perfect addition to anything you want to grill or broil.

**MAKES ABOUT 3 CUPS
(¼ CUP PER SERVING)**

Prep time: 10 minutes

Cook time: 30 minutes

2 tablespoons extra-virgin olive oil

1 onion, chopped

3 garlic cloves, minced

3 cups frozen pitted sweet cherries, chopped

¼ cup honey

¼ cup apple cider vinegar

½ teaspoon sea salt

⅛ teaspoon liquid smoke

1. In a large skillet, heat the olive oil over medium heat. Cook the onion for 5 to 7 minutes until softened and browned. Add the garlic and cook for 30 more seconds until fragrant.

2. Add the cherries, honey, vinegar, salt, and liquid smoke. Bring to a boil and reduce the heat to a simmer. Simmer uncovered for 20 minutes until thickened.

3. Using an immersion blender or in a traditional blender, purée the sauce.

4. Transfer to a jar and store in the refrigerator for up to 5 days, or freeze for up to 2 months.

INGREDIENT TIP: Liquid smoke is made by concentrating the smoke from a wood fire to give food a unique wood-smoked flavor without actually having to smoke it. Look for a brand that does not contain any additional flavorings, for the best quality and to avoid additives.

Per serving: Calories 105; Total fat 2g; Saturated fat 0g; Cholesterol 0mg; Carbs 33g; Fiber 2g; Protein 1g; Sodium 80mg

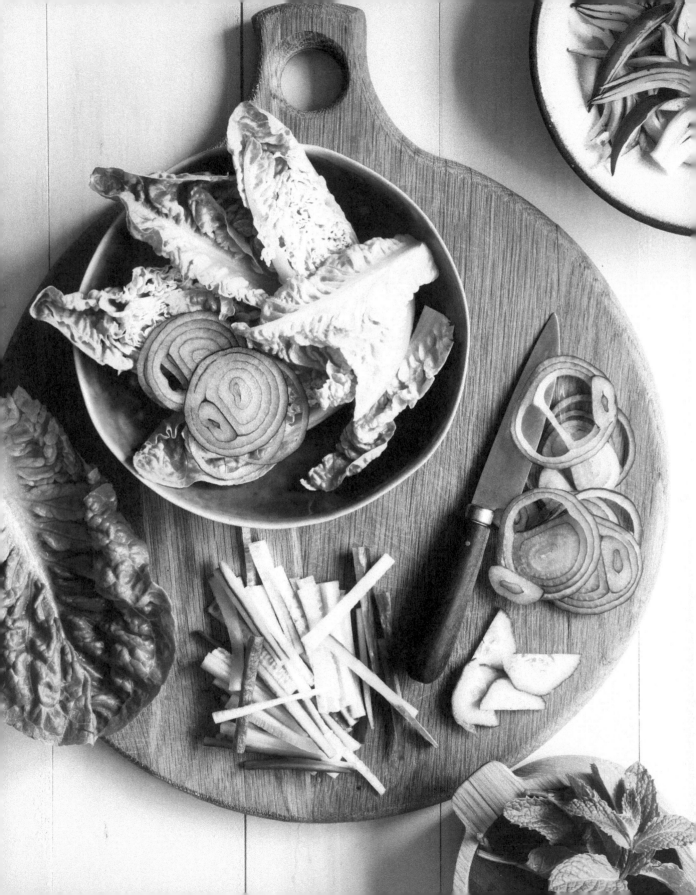

The Dirty Dozen and
Clean Fifteen™

A nonprofit environmental watchdog organization called Environmental Working Group (EWG) looks at data supplied by the U.S. Department of Agriculture (USDA) and the Food and Drug Administration (FDA) about pesticide residues. Each year it compiles a list of the best and worst pesticide loads found in commercial crops. You can use these lists to decide which fruits and vegetables to buy organic to minimize your exposure to pesticides and which produce is considered safe enough to buy conventionally. This does not mean they are pesticide-free, though, so wash these fruits and vegetables thoroughly.

DIRTY DOZEN™

Apples
Celery
Cherries
Grapes
Nectarines
Peaches
Pears
Potatoes
Spinach
Strawberries
Sweet bell peppers
Tomatoes

Additionally, nearly three-quarters of hot pepper samples contained pesticide residues

CLEAN FIFTEEN™

Asparagus
Avocados
Broccoli
Cabbages
Cantaloupes
Cauliflower
Eggplants
Honeydew melons
Kiwis
Mangoes
Onions
Papayas
Pineapples
Sweet corn
Sweet peas (frozen)

Measurement Conversions

VOLUME EQUIVALENTS (LIQUID)

US STANDARD	US STANDARD (OUNCES)	METRIC (APPROXIMATE)
2 tablespoons	1 fl. oz.	30 mL
¼ cup	2 fl. oz.	60 mL
½ cup	4 fl. oz.	120 mL
1 cup	8 fl. oz.	240 mL
1½ cups	12 fl. oz.	355 mL
2 cups or 1 pint	16 fl. oz.	475 mL
4 cups or 1 quart	32 fl. oz.	1 L
1 gallon	128 fl. oz.	4 L

OVEN TEMPERATURES

FAHRENHEIT	CELSIUS (APPROXIMATE)
250°F	120°C
300°F	150°C
325°F	165°C
350°F	180°C
375°F	190°C
400°F	200°C
425°F	220°C
450°F	230°C

VOLUME EQUIVALENTS (DRY)

US STANDARD	METRIC (APPROXIMATE)
⅛ teaspoon	0.5 mL
¼ teaspoon	1 mL
½ teaspoon	2 mL
¾ teaspoon	4 mL
1 teaspoon	5 mL
1 tablespoon	15 mL
¼ cup	59 mL
⅓ cup	79 mL
½ cup	118 mL
⅔ cup	156 mL
¾ cup	177 mL
1 cup	235 mL
2 cups or 1 pint	475 mL
3 cups	700 mL
4 cups or 1 quart	1 L

WEIGHT EQUIVALENTS

US STANDARD	METRIC (APPROXIMATE)
½ ounce	15 g
1 ounce	30 g
2 ounces	60 g
4 ounces	115 g
8 ounces	225 g
12 ounces	340 g
16 ounces or 1 pound	455 g

References

Bisht, Babita, Warren G. Darling, Ruth E. Grossmann, E. Torage Shivapour, Susan K. Lutgendorf, Linda G. Snetselaar, Michael J. Hall, M. Bridget Zimmerman, and Terry L. Wahls. "A Multimodal Intervention For Patients With Secondary Progressive Multiple Sclerosis: Feasibility and Effect on Fatigue." *The Journal of Alternative and Complementary Medicine* 20, no. 5 (2014): 347-55. doi:10.1089/acm.2013.0188.

Blomquist, Caroline, Malin Alvehus, Jonas Burén, Mats Ryberg, Christel Larsson, Bernt Lindahl, Caroline Mellberg, Ingegerd Söderström, Elin Chorell, and Tommy Olsson. "Attenuated Low-Grade Inflammation Following Long-Term Dietary Intervention in Postmenopausal Women With Obesity." *Obesity* 25, no. 5 (2017): 892–900. doi:10.1002/oby.21815.

Calder, Philip C. "Polyunsaturated Fatty Acids and Inflammation." *Prostaglandins, Leukotrienes and Essential Fatty Acids* 75, no. 3 (2006): 197–202. doi:10.1016/j.plefa.2006.05.012.

Capalino, Danielle. *The Microbiome Diet Plan*. Berkeley, California: Rockridge Press, 2017.

Food and Drug Administration. "Final Determination Regarding Partially Hydrogenated Oils (Removing Trans Fat)." *FDA.gov*. 2018. https://www.fda.gov/food/ingredientspackaginglabeling/foodadditivesingredients/ucm449162.htm.

Gordon, Elizabeth. *Allergy-Free Desserts*. Hoboken, New Jersey: John Wiley & Sons, 2010.

Griffith, S. M., J. Fisher, S. Clarke, B. Montgomery, P. W. Jones, J. Saklatvala, and P. T. Dawes, et al. "Do Patients with Rheumatoid Arthritis Established on Methotrexate and Folic Acid 5 Mg Daily Need to Continue Folic Acid Supplements Long Term?" *Rheumatology* 39, no. 10 (2000): 1102–9. doi:10.1093/rheumatology/39.10.1102.

Hodgson, Jonathan M., Natalie C. Ward, Valerie Burke, Lawrence J. Beilin, and Ian B. Puddey. "Increased Lean Red Meat Intake Does Not Elevate Markers of Oxidative Stress and Inflammation in Humans." *The Journal of Nutrition* 137, no. 2 (2007): 363–7. doi:10.1093/jn/137.2.363.

Joachim, David. *Food Substitution Bible*. Toronto: Robert Rose Inc., 2005.

Kumar, K. Kiran, G. Sridhar Reddy, B. V. R. Reddy, P. Chandra Shekar, J. Sumanthi, and K. Lalith Prakash Chandra. "Biological Role of Lectins: A Review." *Journal of Orofacial Sciences* 4, no. 1 (2012): 20–5. doi:10.4103/0975-8844.99883.

Leiba, A., H. Amital, M. E. Gershwin, and Y. Shoenfeld. "Diet and Lupus". *Lupus* 10, no. 3 (2001): 246–8. doi:10.1191/096120301674681790.

Lupus Research Alliance. "What Is Lupus—Lupus Causes, Treatment, and Symptoms." 2018. *Lupus Research*. https://www.lupusresearch.org/understanding-lupus/what-is-lupus.

Maffucci, Ali. *Inspiralized*. New York: Clarkson Potter, 2015.

Pearl, Molly. *Paleo Slow Cooking*. New York: Alpha Books, 2014.

Seymour, Sasha. *Coconut Every Day*. Toronto: Penguin Canada, 2014.

Short, Jenna. *Cooking Allergy-Free*. Newtown, Connecticut: The Taunton Press, 2014.

Takvorian, S. U., J. F. Merola, and K. H. Costenbader. "Cigarette Smoking, Alcohol Consumption and Risk of Systemic Lupus Erythematosus." *Lupus* 23, no. 6 (2014): 537–44. doi:10.1177/0961203313501400.

Whalen, Kristine A., Marjorie L. McCullough, W. Dana Flanders, Terryl J. Hartman, Suzanne Judd, and Roberd M. Bostick. "Paleolithic and Mediterranean Diet Pattern Scores Are Inversely Associated With Biomarkers of Inflammation and Oxidative Balance in Adults." *The Journal of Nutrition* 146, no. 6 (2016): 1217–26. doi:10.3945/jn.115.224048.

Wood, Rebecca. *The New Whole Foods Encyclopedia*. New York: Penguin Books, 2010.

Diet Label Index

Index

Acknowledgments

I would like to thank my family for their ongoing support, particularly my husband, Brian, who let me turn this writing dream into a reality.

Also, an enormous thanks to my virtual support squad, particularly Abbi Perets and Jen Snyder.

About the Author

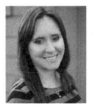 **ANA REISDORF, MS, RD,** is a health and nutrition writer living outside of Nashville, Tennessee, with her husband and two sons. She loves sharing her passion for nutrition through her writing.

Printed in the USA
CPSIA information can be obtained
at www.ICGtesting.com
LVHW052135091223
765798LV00002B/18